Nature's Medicines

D'd you know that *garlic* can reduce fever and lower your blood pressure? That it is effective in treating colds, sinus troubles and throat irritations?

Did you know that *sarsaparilla* is an effective treatment for psoriasis? That it contains the male hormone, testosterone, and that it may ultimately provide a cure for baldness?

Did you know that *ginseng*, the herb more precious than gold, can be grown in radioactive soil? That it can add years of youthful vitality to your life?

Did you know that *ripe cherries* are effective in the treatment of gout and arthritis? That *mint leaves* can be used to cure dandruff?

Did you realise that many ancient herbal cures are accepted today in general medical use, and that modern laboratory tests have proved what the medicine men and witch doctors of other lands and other times have always known?

Nature's Medicines

Richard Lucas

TANDEM
14 Gloucester Road, London SW7

First published in Great Britain by Neville
Spearman Ltd

Published by Universal-Tandem Publishing Co. Ltd, 1972

Made and printed in Great Britain by
Hunt Barnard Printing Ltd., Aylesbury, Bucks.

contents

16. **MISCELLANEOUS HERBS** (*Cont.*):

in Herbs. Medicinal Use of Echinacea. Information on Echinacea from Other Sources. Hawthorn as a Medicine. Modern Research on Hawthorn. How to Distinguish Peppermint from Spearmint. Medicinal Use of Peppermint. Peppermint Remedies. Scientific Research. Medicinal Value. Rose Hips. The Nutritive Properties of Rose Hips. Species of Rose Hips. Acerola Berries. Scientific Investigation of the Acerola Berry. Recent Reports on Vitamin C. The Gentle Action of Slippery Elm. America. Britain. Russia. Research on the Violet.

special notice

It is not the purpose of this book to replace the services of your physician. By all means see a doctor for any condition which requires his services.

Herbs have been used since the beginning of time for medicinal purposes and scientific research is now proving that the plant kingdom contains an abundance of remarkable and valuable healing properties. Millions of dollars a year are being spent by modern drug companies in search of plants that heal.

The botanical materia medica and scientific information given in this book are taken from the writings of doctors, scientific laboratory reports, documents, treatises, and other related sources. No attempt should be made on the part of the reader to use any of this information as a form of treatment without securing the approval of his own medical doctor.

foreword

WHEN MR. LUCAS asked me to write an introduction to his book, I felt flattered as well as apprehensive. His subject matter seemed to me too far removed from my own field of medical practice and scientific research and I was tempted to beg off. But then I started to read the manuscript and soon became absorbed and decidedly fascinated. I learned so much about herbs, plants and plant drugs that I never knew before, that I kept on reading with more and more delight and decided to say so right here at this opportunity.

The introduction to a book is not supposed to be a review. A sharp separation, however, is not always possible. Some of the following lines may therefore seem to be reviewing the contents of Mr. Lucas' volume which they are not meaning to do.

For those physicians who prescribe for their patients other than ready made biologicals that are not of plant origin, Lucas' book appears to be of great value, supplementing a pharmacological reference book that doctors usually have on their desk. For the layman, for whom the book is actually written, it should be a rich source of information, presented in a readable, refreshing and often entertaining form.

Some of the chapters, for instance those on seeds, citrus fruits and on papaya, the "medicine tree," make me wish I could have read them in my student days. They might have helped me at that time to pass examinations in botany and pharmacology. I would not be surprised if Lucas' book would become quite a favorite with medical students, even at this day and age when biological products compete so strongly with pharmaceuticals derived from plants. Reading some of Mr. Lucas' tales makes me think that a new era may be in the making when advanced research may discover new plants and drugs of an as yet unknown application and healing power.

In any event, the scientific data contained in Mr. Lucas' book should not only be of value to the lay reader, but also to the medical and pharmacological student, as well as to the practicing physician and to the druggist.

HARRY BENJAMIN, M.D.

introduction

THE EMPLOYMENT OF herbal remedies as healing agents has been practiced by the forbears of every race and land upon earth. Though separated by the vast expanse of oceans, continents, impenetrable jungles, or deserts, primitive people everywhere possessed a remarkable knowledge of plant medicine. Early mankind, by means of trial and error, accidents, etc., found that certain roots, plants, barks and seeds possessed medicinal properties. These remedies were handed down from one generation to the next. The astonishing fact is that later, when man developed sufficient modes of travel enabling him to establish contact between the various lands, it was learned that in many instances the claims made regarding the particular healing properties of a certain herb found in one area were identical with those claimed for the same herb in another.

A series of medical papyri have been discovered in Egypt over a period of years. One of the longest and most famous, dating from the 2nd century B.C., is called the Papyrus Ebers. These scrolls or documents are reputed to be the world's oldest medical literature. Descriptions of the various ailments suffered by the people of those times were given, and among the herbs employed as remedial agents were myrrh, cummin, peppermint, caraway, fennel, and the oil from olives, to name just a few. Licorice was especially esteemed among the Egyptians, and archaeologists found great quantities of this botanical

13

stored among the fabulous jewelry and art treasures in the 3000 year old tomb of King Tut. Licorice was also one of the first herbs used in China, and is mentioned in their herbal writings as being beneficial to the lives of men in numerous ways.

The earliest Chinese book on medicinal herbs was written by Emperor Shen-ung about 3000 years B.C. In this monumental work, ginseng is regarded as the most potent of the thousands of herbs mentioned. Ginseng is also listed in the ancient medical book of India, the *Atherva Veda,* and described as beneficial in preserving youth and strength.

The Persians, Romans, Greeks, Babylonians, Hebrews, Arabs and other races were all familiar with the use and practice of herbal medicine. In our own country, we are reminded of the fact that the American Indian placed his reliance on the products of forest and field to alleviate his ills. The early colonists were also well-acquainted with the use of herbs, and brought with them to the New World the simple plant remedies that had been used for generations before them. Contact with the Indians gradually added to their medicinal knowledge the qualities and power of many new botanicals gained from the experience of the Red Man's close association with nature. Families freely exchanged this information and almost every individual joined in the search for some new herb or herbs that would prevent or relieve disease.

In many parts of the world today, herbs are still used as remedial agents. The natives in the interior part of Africa possess a knowledge of the medicinal properties of plants that astonishes the European and American. The art of healing in Sumatra consists in the application of the botanicals with which they are expertly skilled. At an early age they become acquainted with the names, qualities and properties of every shrub and herb among the variety with which their country abounds. In Brazil it is said that certain natives are able to run 100 miles at a steady pace, through jungles and over mountains with just a stick of guarana as their only food. Guarana sticks somewhat resemble licorice, while the fruit resembles the hazelnut. According to South American folklore, the stimulating and nutritious quality they claim for guarana was discovered by the Incas 300 years before the white man appeared in the Western hemisphere.

In the vast subcontinent of India, about 2000 plants are listed in the Ayurvedic, Unani and Tibbi systems of medicine, and these herbal remedies provide the most widely used treatment for the people of that area.

Formerly rather contemptuous of herbal folk medicine, modern science is today doing a startling turnabout, and has undertaken a world-wide search for old-time herbal remedies so common to the earlier periods of history as well as the plants currently used among the jungle natives of Africa and Latin America. Botanists and chemists are rereading old books on herbs which give their medicinal uses and properties, while other medical teams are exploring tropical jungles for roots, leaves, barks, and seeds. This search is carried on chiefly by the large drug firms of the United States and Europe.

There are many reasons for the new scientific change of attitude toward herbal medicine. One of the most significant was the discovery of the medicinal value of snakeroot (Rauwolfia) which came from the botanical pharmacopoeia of ancient India. For thousands of years, the natives of India had chewed the root for its calming effects. Ciba Pharmaceutical Company isolated a tranquilizing agent from the root which proved valuable in the treatment of high blood pressure and some types of insanity. This sparked a world-wide search by the various drug firms for other botanicals that may also possess worthwhile medicinal merit.

The results realized so far from this extensive scientific program appear to be very rewarding. The head of one research team has stated that, "We've never had so much success with chemicals invented by man as we're having with plant extracts."

My own interest in herbs began many years ago when I worked on a ranch and noticed that many of the ranchers and their families frequently resorted to the application and use of various wayside "weeds" for the relief of certain ailments. Their apparent effectiveness made a deep impression on me, and later when I moved to the city I began looking around for herb books and other related literature in order to learn as much as possible about the folklore, history, background, and medicinal use of plants. After reading and studying the currently available material I spent several years collecting rare, old, out-of-print medical herbals.

During this period of time, I made the acquaintance of many herbalists, one of whom had been a surgeon as well as an herbalist in China and who had fled his native land when the communists began to take over. Another came from a long line of great Welsh herbalists covering a period of 250 years, while another had been engaged in an exhaustive amount of study and research into the herbal remedies that had been employed among the North American Indians. Others were American, English and German herbalists.

I compiled several large folders containing the information gleaned from these herbalists and then began the task of sorting and filing this material, being careful to note the instances in which they had agreed with one another regarding the medicinal value attributed to a particular herb. This in turn was cross-checked and compared wherever possible with the information contained in the out-of-print medical herbals and currently published material.

This project was an intriguing one, and it was impossible for me to shake the conviction that the plant kingdom could arm the modern physician with a host of valuable healing agents which would give him more power in his fight against disease, if only our scientific research men would concentrate their attention in this direction. I was therefore greatly excited when, in later years I learned that the botanicals were finally being subjected to intensive investigation by scientific teams.

In the attempt to find out just what modern science was discovering, I began contacting numerous laboratories, foundations, pharmacologists, medical doctors, etc., plus digging through modern scientific publications, articles, treatises and other related writings on the subject. The picture gradually fell into place and the sight was an extremely encouraging one.

In writing this book it has been my aim to bring to the attention of the reader, various herbal remedies as they were used down through the ages, and then in the light of modern scientific findings show why these herbal remedies were either completely justified or are demonstrating indications of possibly becoming so. I have also interspersed some of the folklore, romance and history of the herbs, along with a chapter on the mystical plants and the healing properties attributed to some of them. As a further point of interest a chapter is given on herbal preparations for the hair which have been employed by countless people the world over since ages past.

I am deeply grateful to the foundations, authors, publishers, newspapers, magazines, and syndicates who have so generously given me permission to quote or use their material. I also wish to thank Dr. Benjamin for contributing the Foreword. Without the co-operation of all these people, this compilation would not have been possible.

RICHARD LUCAS

I

herbs: our ancient health secret

*All thy garments smell of myrrh, and aloes, and
cassia, out of the ivory palaces, whereby they
have made thee glad.—Psalms 45:8.*

WHAT IS LIFE? In general terms, life may be said to be
the emanation of the vital force of God, a universal
principle that pervades all the works of creation. Health
is an expression of this life principle which shows itself
in symptoms of a sparkling eye, perfect complexion, glossy
hair, buoyant strength and grace of the whole body.
Added to these we find a calm and masterful spirit in the
aged, and a joyous one in the young.

Disease is the opposite of health, and means any de-
parture from the normal condition of the general organism.
It can easily be recognized by the lustreless eye, the
sunken cheek, the parched lips, wracking cough, palpitat-
ing heart, fetid breath, crooked spine, etc.

In health our moments fly with the swiftness of an
arrow and we are scarcely conscious of their rapid exit.
In sickness the contrary is in evidence and our moments
pass in that lingering manner which seems to make our
suffering more acute by reason of the slow belated move-

19

ment of time. To the sick, time does not pass lightly, but with the heavy tread of a giant. Unless all, from the king to the beggar, learn to prize health and avoid disease, death, which is no respecter of persons, will continue to reap an early harvest.

Nature's Way to Perfect Health

With the natural methods available by which health may be preserved or regained, it is astonishing that disease and misery are the general rule, and health and pleasure the exception. Who of the human race can step forth at this moment and say, "I have perfect health. I am now living in that perfect state of nature, or in that perfect mental and physical condition in which God has intended that I should." Scarcely a one.

So marvelous is the gift of health that everyone should try by every means within his power to secure it. This means that some attention must be given to the state of the mind as well as to the state of the body, for mental upset and physical disease go hand in hand. Medical men have stated time and again that excessive negative emotions can cause many serious illnesses. A fit of anger will render the bile acidic and irritating, as well as raise the blood pressure far beyond its normal reading. Many persons have been known to rage so violently that they froth at the mouth and are thrown into spasms. The saliva in such instances has often been found to be poisonous. Sudden fright can cause the heart to stop or the body to tremble violently. Fear has been known to relax the bowels just as surely as though a cathartic had been taken, while in other cases the control of the bladder may be temporarily lost. Intense grief will arrest the secretions of the gastric juices and on occasion has turned the hair white.

Contrast the emotions of love, gratitude, faith, hope, joy and laughter with those of hate, grief, panic, fear, despair and misery. The former are as refreshing to the soul as a gentle rain to the steady grace of a forest. The latter as withering as the fiery blasts of a volcano. The first contributes vital power to the mind, which in turn reactivates the body. The other dissipates, enfeebles, wastes, and seeks to destroy both body and soul together. When we "nourish wrath to keep it warm" we inject venom into a heart that was created in love. That anger which "dwells only in the bosom of fools" should have no inheritance in the bosom of the wise and thoughtful of our race. Fretting, scolding and faultfinding not only aggravate all the evils of the world but greatly multiply them. We thus dissipate our best talents and energies, and render life a curse instead of a blessing. We stamp infirmities on the body which hurry us to an early grave. Therefore it is imperative that everyone make an endeavor to learn the art of adapting themselves to the invariable laws of God's universe, which they cannot successfully oppose, or in any respect alter, without paying the price of the "uttermost farthing." To constantly cherish and maintain an even, cheerful and hopeful spirit is one of the prime requisites to good health.

The Medicine of Primitive Man

As to our bodily needs, there has always been a belief shared by a great number of people in many lands, that an all-wise Providence has supplied man, in the great natural laboratories of forest and field, with plants capable of serving his every requirement. Reflecting upon the remote past, we find that it was both natural and sensible that man, having found in plants the source of his food supply when in health, should again turn to nature when illness assailed him.

Primitive man did not possess intelligence as we know it today. He was not equipped with the mentality which would enable him to probe into the bowels of the earth, extracting a variety of substances, and putting them through complex processes by which they would finally emerge as synthetic drugs. If primitive man was to survive and evolve, then his medicine had to be as obvious and simple as his food. We know that he was not wrong in following his instinct, for in the plants, shrubs, roots, and barks he found effective remedies for his daily needs.

Man has now evolved to a point of expressing and enjoying a profound intelligence, and realizes that he is God's highest creation, empowered with dominion over the lesser forms of life. Yet this "highest" creation is suffering from dreaded diseases and all the multitude of ills that can befall the human body, while the lesser, the animal life, still abounds in strength and vitality, and frolics carefree upon the bosom of nature. Like the prodigal son, man has overlooked and disregarded that which is near at hand, and has wandered afar in search of inferior substitutes. And once again, like the prodigal son he must "rise up" and return to the house of the Father . . . the ways of God and His laws. Nothing has changed, and the green plants, drawing from the rays of the sun that precious something which sustains life and without which man would perish and the earth become a barren waste, are the same yesterday, today, and forever. The guiding light that will lead man back from the confused world of his own making is the Holy Bible.

Herbs and the Bible

The general term *herb* or *herbs* is mentioned 37 times in Sacred Scripture, and there is constant and repeated mention of the botanicals by their names. For example:

Is there no balm in Gilead; is there no physician there? why then is not the health of the daughter of my people recovered?—Jer. 8:22. Go up into Gilead, and take balm, O virgin, the daughter of Egypt: in vain shalt thou use many medicines; for thou shalt not be cured.—Jer. 46:11.

Balm of Gilead is a small tree native to Arabia. A resinous substance is obtained by making incisions in the tree, and is still sold today extensively in Arabia and other Asiatic countries. When first exuded, the substance is white, but later turns to a golden color and resembles honey in consistency. The buds of the tree are used as a medicinal remedy for disorders of the lungs, stomach, and kidneys. They are also prepared as an ointment and used for rheumatic or gouty pains.

And Isaiah said, Take a lump of figs. And they took it and laid it on the boil, and he recovered.— 2 Kings 20:7.

Among the Hebrews the fig tree was associated with the vine as a symbol of peace and plenty. Figs are still used as medicine in many lands throughout the world today. In Bavaria they are cooked in milk for use in treating ulcerated gums. Among the Hindus the milky juice of the tree is given to relieve toothache, while in America the juice is used in treatment of ringworm and warts. Figs heated and cut open are placed on gum boils to draw out the matter. For pulmonary complaints they are boiled in barley water.

Instead of the thorn shall come up the fir tree, and instead of the briar shall come up the myrtle tree: and it shall be to the Lord for a name, for an everlasting sign that shall not be cut off.—Isa. 55:13.

Myrtle signified the promise and bounty of God to the Jews. In ancient times its beautiful foliage served as wreaths and other ornamentations for the adornment of heroes, in the performance of religious rites, and as an emblem of civil authority. In some parts of Greece its evergreen quality was symbolic of immortality. Myrtle is used as a remedy for rheumatism, internal ulcers, and dysentery. The leaves are employed for making a gargle and as a preparation for perfume.

The mysterious *manna* that fell from heaven, and which has puzzled Bible authorities and students to this day, is believed by many to have been a type of plant substance.

> Then the Lord said unto Moses, Behold, I will rain bread from heaven for you; and the people shall go out and gather a certain rate every day, that I may prove them, whether they walk in my law, or no.— Ex. 16:4. And when the children of Israel saw it, they said one to another, It is manna: for they wist not what it was.—Ex. 16:15.

The word *manna* means, "What is this?" The substance called manna today is the saccharine juice of different plants or trees (the Tamarisks) which seeps through a natural or induced rupture of the bark. The Tamarisk tree and its properties were highly valued by the Arabs. Their renowned physician, Avicenna, in his *System of Medicine,* recommended its different parts as valuable healing agents. This tree is believed to have some connection with the Biblical manna; however, the conditions under which the "bread of heaven" was found, and the properties it contained, were very different from any of the known mannas. In spite of this difference, the description of the Biblical manna definitely suggests a plant substance: *And the man-na was as coriander seed, and the colour thereof as the colour of bdellium*—Nu. 11:7. We are also told that it tasted like freshly-expressed oil from the olive and like wafers made with honey.

Interwoven throughout the mystical and beautiful Song of Solomon are the herbs, spices, and gardens which provided the perfect setting for this song of love. *Thy plants are an orchard of pomegranates, with pleasant fruits; camphire, with spikenard, Spikenard and saffron; calamus and cinnamon, with all trees of frankincense; myrrh and aloes, with all the chief spices:—S.S. 4:13, 14.* When the Lord appeared to Solomon in a dream and told him to ask whatever he desired, Solomon requested an understanding heart. This greatly pleased the Lord and He replied: *Behold, I have done according to thy words: lo, I have given thee a wise and an understanding heart; so that there was none like thee before thee, neither after thee shall any arise like unto thee.—I Ki. 3:12.* Rulers of the earth came to seek advice and counsel from this great man of Biblical times who had received the gift of wisdom from God.

The writing of 39 books is attributed to King Solomon. One of these was an herbal, giving the botanical remedies for every disease. This priceless book was held in a sacred temple in Jerusalem, but was destroyed during the fall of the ancient city of the Jews, by the Roman General Titus. Among the valuable books in the great library of Alexandria was a second copy of the remarkable herbal of Solomon, until this too, was destroyed.

The thread of truth regarding the use of botanicals and the high esteem in which they were held runs throughout the New Testament as well as the Old. In St. Mark 14:3, we read: *And being in Bethany in the house of Simon the leper, as he sat at meat, there came a woman having an alabaster box of ointment of spikenard very precious; and she brake the box, and poured it on his head.* Spikenard is an aromatic plant. The ancients gathered the roots for use in preparing valuable perfumes which were used at celebrated feasts and in the baths of the wealthy. Spikenard was, of course, also used as medicine. Sacred Scripture tells us that our Lord commanded His disciples that wherever the gospel was preached throughout the world that some mention be made of the good work this woman had done to Him. It may be pointed out that it would be impossible for the disciples to obey this command without also mentioning the herb, spikenard. This indicates a desire on the part of the Master that the disciples spread and immortalize the powerful truth of His blessed herbs as well as the tribute to the kindness of the woman.

The following familiar passage is taken from St. Matthew 2:11: *and when they had opened their treasures, they presented unto him gifts; gold, and frankincense, and myrrh.* Frankincense was burned both by the Egyptians and Jews in their religious rites. The odor of incense was believed to center the mind on devotion, produce an elevated mental state and in some way affect the psychic body. Modern man may frown upon such beliefs as being entirely superstitious, yet it cannot be denied that certain odors do cause powerful reactions in people. Some odors can nauseate, cause headache, upset the stomach, and bring about a state of illness. The aroma of certain foods can start the saliva flowing before the food actually enters the mouth. A whiff of pepper can trigger a reaction of sneezing.

Frankincense is still used today as an incense, and in Egypt the gum is chewed to sweeten the breath. It is also an excellent fixative in heavy Oriental perfumes.

Myrrh was regarded as one of the most precious of nature's products. It was probably valued above all others as an incense ingredient and was burned on altars, mixed with benzoin, during the time of Moses and before.

Hyssop is mentioned in the Gospel of St. John: *After this, Jesus knowing that all things were now accomplished, that the scripture might be fulfilled, saith, I thirst. Now there was set a vessel full of vinegar: and they filled a sponge with vinegar, and put it upon hyssop, and put it to his mouth.—John 19:28, 29.* Hyssop was the symbol of purification from sin. In the old days, the early herbalists and country folk used hyssop leaves on fresh wounds to protect against infections and promote healing. Doctors thought that this was sheer superstitious nonsense until they discovered that the mold that produces penicillin grows on hyssop leaves!

The Law of Healing

Now as we have seen, in primitive man it was essential that his medicine be both obvious and easily obtainable. Once God had established His law of healing it was established forever. But to keep pace with man's ever-expanding intelligence the law had to be held before his eyes at each stage of his growth, whether yesterday, today, or a thousand years hence. To meet this requirement it was written with an immortal hand in an immortal book —*The Holy Bible.*

> *And God said, Behold, I have given you every herb bearing seed, which is upon the face of all the earth, and every tree, in the which is the fruit of a tree yielding seed; to you it shall be for meat.*— Gen. 1:29
>
> *. . . and the fruit thereof shall be for meat, and the leaf thereof for medicine.*—Ezk. 47:12.

II

how ancient herbs become modern medicine

. . . and the leaves of the tree were for the healing of the nations.—Rev. 22:2.

TRY AS IT may, modern medicine cannot quite shake itself entirely free from the ancient womb from which it sprang. Those who have traced the symbol of the modern physician, that of a staff with two snakes coiled around it, have found its origin in the "Greek God of Medicine." This was the title given to Aesculapius, the ancient Greek physician whose healing powers were considered so miraculous that mysterious legends surrounded his life, and after death he was raised to the stature of a God. Many healing temples were erected in his honor, and his statue, depicting him with a staff around which a snake was coiled, was placed in each temple. The snake, according to mythology, was supposed to have a supreme knowledge of the healing power of herbs and is shown in the statue with an herb in its mouth. One of the daughters of Aesculapius, Hygeia, became deified as a Goddess of Health, and it is from her name that we get the word *hygiene*. His other daughter, whose success in using herbal remedies for the cure of diseases won for her the deification of "Goddess of Medicine," was named *Panacea,* the word which is still in use today, meaning "cure-all."

The familiar sign *Rx,* which is generally found in the upper left-hand corner of the modern prescription, has been traced to the pagan symbol for Jupiter (♃). It has been said that the ancient practice of placing this symbol at the head of prescriptions was instituted in the time of Nero, when the Christians were being brutally persecuted, to indicate an allegiance of the physician to the State religion of Rome. It meant, "Take thou in the name of Jupiter." We are told that the ancients employed the Greek word *Physis,* meaning the natural constitution, to signify pharmacy and sorcery, and that in this way those who taught and practiced the healing art came to be known as "physicians."

The code of medical ethics known as the Hippocratic Oath is still taken today by graduating students in many medical schools. Hippocrates, the Father of Medicine, lived from 460 to 377 B.C., and was one of the most observing and industrious men who ever lived. He was the first to conceive the idea of diagnosis and also exercised great care in regulating the diet of persons afflicted with acute diseases. Wounds were treated with the view of guarding against undue loss of blood. Herbs, diet, baths, fresh air, massage, rest and quiet formed the bulk of his treatments, and he made his followers swear on oath that they would give no poisonous remedies to their patients. Between three and four hundred plants are mentioned in what are known as the Hippocratic Writings.

The Search for Ancient Cures

It appears that the modern healing art is not only clothed in signs, symbols and traditions of the ancients, but the vital power, that of ancient medicine itself, is beginning to penetrate the heart of modern medication. A very enlightening and interesting article was published in *Popular Mechanics* (April 1960) entitled, "In Search of Plants That Cure," by James Joseph. The article tells us that medical experts armed with walkie-talkies, mobile labs and aqualungs are searching the four corners of the earth, seas, and even the American back yard for medicinal plants. A top researcher comments: "We've come full circle. Back in the 1800's, fully 80 percent of the medicines were plant derived. Gradually, researchers turned more and more to chemicals, both organic and inorganic. Today, half the curatives in the average family's medicine cabinet are products of somebody's test tube. And only 30 percent are plant based. Now, almost out of desperation, we're going back to nature—back to plants. For good as the test tube is, it hasn't cured man's greatest cripplers—arthritis, heart trouble, insanity, asthma and cancer."

Five-Million-Dollar Gamble

The article goes on to say that the drug companies were gambling five million dollars in that year alone to outfit safaris because they believed that, "there may be more fact than fiction in witch doctor remedies, medical folklore and tribal cure-all."

Just how the researchers know where to look for possible healing plants, we are told, is often started by a rumor somewhat like the following: "From the milk-white sap of a jungle herb, a witch doctor has been extracting a potion that cures insanity." When the medical expert finally locates the witch doctor and comes to terms, he recognizes the plant he is shown as one that grows in almost every back yard in America. The jungle plant searcher immediately radios his employer, a pharmaceutical company and refers to the plant by code name. We are informed that the message states: "Investigate plant L57-67 . . . as possible cure for insanity."

The article mentions that Dr. Saleem A. Farag of the

College of Medical Evangelists, Loma Linda, California, recently brought back 80 plants that had been used regularly by the Ha tribe of East Africa as medicine: "We're literally leaving no plant unturned," Dr. Farag says, and adds further that, "Our search is reaching into every American back yard. There's just no telling about a plant, until it has been squeezed dry of its secrets."

The Witch Doctors' Remedies

The article states that more than 1000 plant detectives are searching five continents and the seas for medicinally promising plants, and relates some of the interesting ways in which plants were "discovered" accidentally. For example, we are told that the brother of an African foreman had a severe toothache and a U. S. dentist, after examination, said that the tooth would have to be pulled. Instead of consenting, the patient went to a "witch doctor" (actually an authentic practitioner of plant medicine). Within minutes, the patient was cured. The amazed dentist drove for three days in his jeep over primitive trails in search of the fantastic healer. When he found the native physician and managed to get him to relate his cure, he immediately sent the information back to the States, describing the plant and using the code number, F57-11. The cure was reported as being accomplished by the following method: "The native doctor filled half a gourd with water and covered it with the other half in whose top he'd drilled a hole. Over the hole he placed three small sticks dipped in animal fat and rolled in the seeds taken from plant F57-11. He ignited the sticks and allowed them—and the seeds—to burn slowly. The medicating smoke was directed to the offending tooth through a straw. Complete relief was obtained."

The article mentions a startling "incident" which occurred in "nearby Baja California." A scientist's guide who was a native of Mexico cut himself severely by accident. The flow of blood apparently did not upset the guide in the least as he calmly walked over to a shrub, picked a few leaves and placed them on the wound. The bleeding stopped almost immediately. We are informed that, "no drug known today comes close to duplicating this feat."

Dr. Farag reports a frustrating experience as he tells of a mission doctor who, "diagnosed a tribesman's illness as schizophrenia, a mental disorder that afflicts millions the world over." It seems that a native healer treated the patient and returned him to apparent sanity within a short period of time. We can well imagine the astonishment experienced by the mission doctor, as we are told that modern medicine has no sure cure for this illness.

Accompanied by a guide, Dr. Farag began his search for the remarkable native healer. The witch doctor was found drunk with "a gourd of home-brewed banana beer in one hand and violence in his eyes." Any attempt on the part of Dr. Farag to get him to release his secret was useless as the native practitioner refused point blank. Dr. Farag, we are told, tried again about a week later but the witch doctor who apparently had a violent temper, ranted and absolutely refused any offer of money or his usual fee, which is a cow, to give out the precious information.

Dr. Farag says, "The thing haunts me. We know that one patient was cured by whatever it was the fellow used. And, though we always take with a proverbial grain of salt even the most locally renowned of native cures, you never know until you've put a plant through the research wringer."

Investigating Natural Plant Cures for Cancer

The article also reports that, "Natural plant cures for cancer, long scoffed at by researchers, are being seriously investigated by the National Cancer Institute." Dr. Jonathan Hartwell of the Institute, we are told, was busy researching through ancient literature, some of which dates back 3500 years, such as the Egyptian medical scrolls. At the time the article was written, he had turned up two promising plants, the juniper tree and the American mandrake. Both these plants appeared to destroy cancer cells in test animals.

We are informed that Dr. Mervin Hardinge at California's College of Medical Evangelists, backed by a grant from the U.S. Public Health Service, was attempting a tremendous job. The doctor and his staff intended to dissect every plant that grows in California in hopes of discovering medicinal properties. Out of 1500 plants that had been taken apart in three years, at least a half dozen showed definite effects upon cancer in laboratory animals.

Dr. Hardinge reported that the "most promising" cancer plant he had been testing was a native of Oregon. He explained that, "One of our faculty members was vacationing in Oregon and brought this plant back—partly on a hunch, partly because local folks had for years been using it as a medicine. Tests show it to be highly active. In fact, it shows real signs of inhibiting the growth of some cancer cells. It'll take years, perhaps, to prove its worth—and safety—for human patients. But right now we're putting the plant to the medical test with better than anticipated results."

The article tells us that University of Arizona botanists are on the same trail, searching every desert plant for a possible cure for cancer.

Dr. Alfred Taylor, heading a research team of the University of Texas, states: "We've never had as much success with chemicals invented by man as we're having with plant extracts."

Medical Plants Often Discovered by Accident

The informative article mentions a few of the plant "discoveries" that have been made into modern medicines.

North Chicago's big Abbott Laboratories announced discovery of a drug which is effective against hardening of the arteries (arteriosclerosis) in 1957, and the basis for the new drug was ". . . oil pressed from the seeds of the East Indian safflower, a thistlelike herb whose American relative is the common garden aster."

Snakeroot (Rauwolfia) was another plant which yielded its secret to the modern lab, according to the article, which tells us that it has been said that even Gandhi used the Indian plant, Rauwolfia, and dipped it into his teas for its calming effects. It also points out the fact, known to almost every herbalist, that the roots had been chewed for 30 centuries among Indian and African natives to alleviate nervous depression and adds that "no less than one million Indians regularly used the herb."

We are told that it was not until 1931 that Western researchers took serious notice of the plant, and when they did, it was not until 1952 that they uncovered its potent source found mostly in the root, and which is called *reserpine*. This "discovery" resulted in the modern tranquilizer. A drug company executive commented, "We finally figured that one million Indians couldn't be wrong."

We are also informed that curare, long used as a poison on the arrows of the jungle savages of the Amazon, was "discovered" by modern science only in 1938. Curare is now considered a "top rate anesthetic (particularly in abdominal surgery), a muscle relaxer and a 'standard' for treating some victims of mental disorders, including manic-depressives."

The extract from the leaves of the foxglove plant used in the treatment of certain types of heart trouble was an old time European folk remedy. This extract is commonly known as digitalis.

Seaweed-derived iodine, an old Polynesian antiseptic, is a staple in your medicine cabinet and mine.

All were "discovered" often by accident, when skeptical researchers decided to test the truth of an ancient remedy.

The "Most Wanted" Plant Remedies

In conclusion, we are informed by the article that medical researchers want information on any plant with a local record for curing. "The fact that plant X is a generally accepted home remedy puts it on the plant hunter's 'most wanted' list." The reader is given details, suggestions and advice on how to identify the plant, submit his notes to medical researchers, etc. He is further assured that it isn't necessary to try to find a new plant. "The fact is that almost every plant in your garden has, one time or another, been used—and prescribed—as a local remedy, if only to treat sunburn. What's more, it's a safe bet that growing within a dozen miles of your home, city dweller though you may be, is a plant which, incredible as it may seem, has escaped the botanists."

Now as the years drift by, it appears as though little or no further mention is made of the results of such research and many people begin to wonder whether or not the whole thing proved impractical. We must remember that the scientific approach is a complicated one, one that takes time, patience, and tireless effort. The article reveals the fact that in the 1850s only 6000 of the 350,-000 plants that are known to exist today had been examined and classified, and further states that some 4000 species that are "new" to the botanist today, are added each year to the list. The article also gives us a good idea of just what the further scientific approach entails:

Herbs in the Laboratory

In the laboratory, scientists set to work with a phalanx of research tools: *grinders,* which reduce the plant's parts to the consistency of milled wheat; *chemi-*

cals, including acids, which dissolve out or separate the raw plant extract, which may contain upwards of 200 substances, known and unknown; *electrostatic machines,* designed to isolate substances electrically; a *counter-current distributor* whose complex net of glass tubes separates compounds which are soluble; and finally, an *infrared spectrophotometer* which, when a plant's vital and pure ingredients are found, double-checks them for purity.

It's a little like panning for gold—for a golden, perhaps revolutionary, medical discovery. The plant's raw substances, like raw pay dirt, are chemically dissolved until every *known* substance is washed away. Finally, there remains only the pure extract, perhaps a chemical or crystal never before put to the medical test.

Then of course come the lengthy experiments with laboratory animals. In the end, if the new extract is proven ineffective or harmful it is discarded and the entire process is repeated with another promising plant. This gives us a very good idea why it may be many years before we hear of a new scientifically developed plant formula. That science is continuing its plant research with an ever-increasing pace cannot for a moment be doubted, as more recent information states that the drug companies are spending around 25 million dollars a year for this research, as against the 5 million quoted back in 1960 when the article was written.

Scientific Research on Plants Used by the American Indians

A report published in *Drug Topics,* March 23, 1964, mentions that a three-year grant of $125,700 was awarded to the Oregon State University School of Pharmacy by the U. S. Public Health Service for a study of the plants of the Pacific Northwest. The proposed study calls for special attention to be directed to plants found in the Warm Springs Indian reservation to determine whether plants used by the Indians over the centuries have any real therapeutic value.

According to the article, the program is scheduled to be directed by Dr. Leo A. Sciuchetti, professor of pharmacognosy, and includes authorities in medicine, pharmacy and botany at various institutions and universities throughout the country.

The First Year of the Project

During the first year about 20 plants believed to have therapeutic value would be collected and identified by Dr. David H. French, professor of anthropology at Reed College, Portland. Dr. French is an expert on the nutritional and medicinal uses of wild plants employed in the Warm Springs area by the Indians. Some of the plants scheduled to be collected and studied are wild peony, bitter cherry, wild columbine, ocean spray, poison hemlock, shelf fungus, creek dogwood and alum root. We are told that men of science believe that these plants and others may contain medicinal properties which would prove valuable as sedatives, antibiotics, astringents, pain killers, tranquilizers, and in the treatment of venereal disease, diabetes, heart disease and nervous system conditions.

According to Dr. Sciuchetti there has been no intensive screening of the plants of the Pacific Northwest for medicinal value although some of the plant species have been studied. He states further that "the climate and topography of the area are suited to an abundance of plants ranging from temperate coastal to alpine types."

Second and Third Year Studies

During the following two years of research, plant material will be collected by Dr. Kenton Chambers, Oregon State University associate professor of botany. It will be gathered from the Coast range and coastal areas of Oregon, and from the higher ranges of the Cascades and Eastern Oregon. The plant materials will be prepared and extracted for study by the Oregon State University pharmacognosy department. The charge of screening all plant material for medicinal activity will go to Dr. Rob S. McCutcheon, professor of pharmacognosy. He will make a detailed study of plants which indicate possible properties in treatment of heart, nervous, and insulin-like activity.

Dr. Philip Catalfomo, assistant professor of pharmacognosy at Oregon State University, will test the plants indicating anti-bacterial activity. Dr. Jonathan L. Hartwell of the National Institute of Health, Bethesda, Maryland, will determine the anti-tumor activity in plants, while the study of plants indicating tranquilizing effects will be undertaken by Dr. Joseph P. Buckley, professor of pharmacology at the University of Pittsburgh. The pharmacognosy and pharmaceutical departments at Oregon State University will work jointly on the chemical identification of active compounds, under the direction of Dr. H. Wayne Schultz, assistant professor of pharmaceutical chemistry.

Dr. Sciuchetti credits new methods of extraction and evaluation with stimulating an ever-increasing interest in plants throughout the world. He feels that the research of medicinal plants as a new source of drugs is "wide open," and points out that plant screening programs are now being carried on in the Southwest, Ohio, and Mexico.

For Every Disease an Herbal Remedy?

It can be clearly seen that we are steadily gaining scientific proof that man's medicine is exactly where the Bible has always said that it was—in the plant kingdom.

From the many facts existing, we may well believe that there is not a single disease in man that may not have its remedy or cure in some herb or other, if we but knew *which* plant and where to find it. For who has not often seen, not only our own domestic animals, but many of the untamed creatures of forest, field, and sky, seek out some one particular herb when laboring under sickness or some derangement of its organism? Nature has, of course, wisely implanted a definite instinct in these creatures, in order to serve for its health or restoration to health from disease. In man, however, such instinct is not so plainly marked, but to him has been given reason and judgment and a disposition to investigate the laws and mysteries of creation in order to secure his own highest health and perfection. As the proverb says, "There are sermons in stones, and books in running brooks;" so do we behold volumes of wisdom in all the herbal kingdom—every emerald and variegated leaf, in every tinted blossom. In *all,* there is a voiceless language, eternally singing significant psalms in praise of "Him who doeth all things well."

The ancients, Indians, and simple country folk heard the voiceless strains and lifted their hearts in thanksgiving to God for His great mercy and accepted His prescription without question. He honored their faith by healing them. For years such people have been bitterly criticized, laughed at, and sometimes even pitied for their "stupidity." But it is to these same people who held on to their faith in God's herbal remedies with a tenacity that defies the imagination, to whom the world now pays its belated homage.

III

the bulb with miracle healing powers

*We remember the fish, which we did eat in Egypt
freely; the cucumbers, and the melons, and the
leeks, and the onions, and the garlick:*
—Numbers: 11:5.

MIRACULOUS HEALING POWER appears to exist in common
garlic. Research shows that for over 5000 years it has
been used to cure many ailments that are being studied
today in modern scientific laboratories. The Babylonians
knew of its curative power as early as 3000 B.C. Garlic
was highly honored and esteemed in ancient Egypt, and
thousands of slaves working on the great Cheops pyramid
were fed garlic daily. In ancient times, the soldiers relied
on the bulb to give them added strength in battle. The
Phoenicians and Vikings carried large amounts of garlic
with them on their sea voyages. The wandering Israelites
bemoaned the fact that they had no more garlic as they
once had enjoyed so freely when in Egypt.

In Bulgaria there is a surprising number of people who
reach the age of 100 who are still active and working. In

that country it is a common practice among the ordinary people to chew garlic regularly.

The Medicinal Use of Garlic in Early Times

The Chinese, Greeks, Romans, Hindus, Egyptians and Babylonians all claimed that garlic cured intestinal disorders, flatulence, worms, infections of the respiratory system, skin diseases, wounds and the symptoms of aging. Aristophanes regarded the juice as a restorer of masculine vigor. Pliny stated that garlic had "very powerful properties" and added that even its odor drove away serpents and scorpions.

Dioscorides, a Greek physician of the second century who accompanied the Roman armies as their official physician, specified garlic for all lung and intestinal disorders occurring among the soldiers. He also considered the herb as a vermifuge. Hippocrates classified garlic as a sudorific and added that it was also effective as a laxative and diuretic. Mohammed said that when garlic is "applied on the sting of the scorpion or the bite of the viper it produces favorable results." Galen cited it as an antidote for poison.

During the Middle Ages when the horrible plagues raged through Europe, it is said that those who ate garlic daily were not infected. Contagion was purportedly held in check by disinfecting the crowded burial grounds with the powerful herb.

In Marseilles, a garlic-vinegar preparation known as the *Four Thieves* was credited with protecting many of the people when a plague struck that city (1722). Some say that the preparation originated with four thieves who confessed that they used it with complete protection against the plague while they robbed the bodies of the dead. Others claim that a man named Richard Forthave developed and sold the preparation, and that the "medicine" was originally referred to as Forthave's. However, with the passing of time, his surname became corrupted to *Four Thieves*.

Garlic and the Old-Time Family Doctor

Garlic was highly valued among the materia medica of the former "family physician." From the *Home-Book of Health* by John Gunn, M.D. (1878), we find the following:

> Garlic is a stimulant, diuretic and expectorant, and applied to the skin, rubefacient, that is, it will produce a blister. The medical uses of garlic are very numerous, it being recommended by some as a valuable expectorant in Consumption and all Affections of the Lungs; by some as an important diuretic in Dropsies, and again by others as a remedy for Fevers, especially of the Intermittent type. It is generally considered a good remedy for Worms, and is often given to children for that purpose. It is an excellent remedy in Nervous and Spasmodic Coughs, Hoarseness, and the like; and may be given in the form of a syrup, tincture, or in substances; but the best way to use it when fresh, is to express the juice, and mix it either with syrup or some other proper vehicle . . .

W. T. Fernie, M.D., wrote an account of the bulb in his book *Herbal Simples*, 1897. Here are a few excerpts:

> The bulb, consisting of several combined cloves, is stimulating, antispasmodic, expectorant, and diuretic. Its active properties depend on an essential oil which may be readily obtained by distillation. A medicinal tincture is made (H.) with spirit of wine, of which from ten to twenty drops may be taken in water several times a day. Garlic proves useful in asthma, whooping-cough and other spasmodic affections of the chest. For an adult, one or more cloves may be eaten at a time. The odour of the bulb is very diffusible,

even when it is applied to the soles of the feet its odour is exhaled by the lungs.

Dr. Bowles, a noted English physician of former times, made use of garlic with much success as a secret remedy for asthma. He concocted a preserve from the boiled cloves with vinegar and sugar, to be kept in an earthen jar. The dose was a bulb or two with some of the syrup, each morning when fasting. The pain of rheumatic parts may be much relieved by simply rubbing them with cut garlic.

Scientific Research on Garlic

Through laboratory experiments, an enormous amount of scientific interest in garlic has resulted. Reports from all over the world are slowly confirming many of the empirical beliefs in the healing power of this humble herb. From the results of experiments made by Rico (Compt. rend. soc. biol., 1926, 95, 1597), garlic has received some scientific support as an anthelmintic. In Germany in 1931, Fusaganger and Becher found that garlic was effective against intestinal putrefaction. French scientist Pouillard found that garlic causes a decided drop in blood pressure. Amano and Kitagawa of Japan reported in 1935 that garlic possesses antiseptic properties which are effective against the typhoid bacillus. It is said that Dr. Albert Schweitzer employed garlic in typhus and cholera.

During World War II, thousands of tons of garlic were purchased by the British government for treating the wounds of soldiers. Not one case of septic poisoning occurred among those treated with garlic. In Brazil in 1948, a group of physicians reported the successful use of a garlic extract among more than 400 patients stricken with intestinal infections. Dehydrated garlic has been employed for its carminative effect in various functional gastrointestinal disorders (Rev. Gastroenterol., 1949, 16, 411).

Investigations by Russian scientists have made garlic

oil so popular in their country that it is referred to as *Russian Penicillin*. Russian clinics and hospitals use garlic almost entirely in the form of volatile extracts. These are not taken by mouth, but are vaporized and inhaled.

Garlic and High Blood Pressure

From experiments on both animals and humans, De-Bray and Loeper (Bull. soc. méd., 1921, 37, 1032) found that garlic tincture causes a decided drop in blood pressure in cases of hypertension. Consistent reductions in blood pressure in 80 cases of hypertension treated with garlic was reported by Ortner in Germany in 1929. Guillon and DeSeze, in 1930, also reported that garlic was effective in relieving high blood pressure. Schlesinger cited a drop in pressure after 15 days' treatment with garlic.

G. Piotrowski, visiting lecturer and member of the faculty of medicine at the University of Geneva, wrote an article in a European publication, *Praxis,* for July 1, 1948, in which he relates his experiences with the use of garlic on "about a hundred patients." [1]

He reports that in 40 percent of the cases he obtained a drop of at least 2 cm. in blood pressure. During this experiment, he took every precaution to make certain that the drop was due to the administration of garlic and nothing else. In treating patients with high blood pressure, Dr. Piotrowski begins by administering fairly large doses of garlic which are gradually diminished over a period of three weeks. He then continues with smaller doses for the balance of the treatment. (He does not say how long he continues the treatment with the smaller doses but we suppose he means until the patient's blood pressure is normal.) He reports that the subjective symptoms

[1] J. I. Rodale, *The Health Finder,* Rodale Books, Inc., Emmaus, Pennsylvania, 1954.

of dizziness, angina-like pains, headaches, and backaches began to disappear in three to five days after garlic treatment began. The patients were all allowed to go about their daily work, so inactivity or bed rest did not have a chance to influence the results. They claimed that they could think more clearly and perform their jobs better.

Dr. Piotrowski also mentions that the expected drop of 2 cm. in blood pressure generally takes place after about a week of treatment. He states further that it appears as though neither the age nor the blood pressure reading of any particular patient can enable one to predict the results, for apparently the good results are not obtained just because the patient is young or because his blood pressure is not too high. He concludes by recommending that many more medical doctors include garlic therapy in treating hypertensive patients.

Garlic and Tuberculosis

At the beginning of the century, Dr. W. C. Minchin, an English physician practicing in Ireland, wrote many letters and articles to the *Lancet* and other British publications on the subject of garlic.[2]

At that time, tuberculosis was the number one killer, and Dr. Minchin was in charge of a large tuberculosis ward at Kells Hospital in Dublin. He was getting remarkable results with his treatment of this dreaded disease. At Dr. Minchin's request, several physicians sent their own tubercular patients to his hospital. While undergoing treatment, these patients were frequently visited by their own doctors who expressed profound astonishment at their improvement and seriously contemplated just what kind of method Dr. Minchin could possibly be using. They did not once suspect that he was employing com-

[2] *Ibid.*

mon ordinary garlic. He administered this as an inhalant, as internal medicine, and as compresses and ointments.

Physicians all over the world were intensely interested in his published letters and articles, and wrote to him telling of their own experiences with the employment of garlic medication. They also told him of the various ways in which they found that many individuals had been using garlic in their own homes for colds, intestinal and digestive disorders, boils, coughs, etc.

Dr. M. W. McDuffie of the Metropolitan Hospital in New York was experimenting with tuberculosis at about the same time as Dr. Minchin's papers were being published in England.[3] In the *North American Journal of Homeopathy* for May 1914, an article appeared by Dr. McDuffie called "Tuberculosis Treatment." In it he tells of 56 different treatments that were used on 1082 patients. These treatments covered everything from hydrochloric acid to chest surgery, to garlic. Of the 56 treatments employed, he says:

> Garlic is the best individual treatment found to get rid of germs and we believe same to be a specific for the tubercle bacillus and for tubercular processes no matter what part of the body is affected, whether skin, bones, glands, lungs or special parts . . . Thus nature, by diet, rest, and exercise, baths, climate, and garlic, furnishes sufficient and specific treatment for the medical aspects of this disease.

Garlic and Intestinal Disorders

Due to modern laboratories it can now be shown exactly how garlic works on germs and proves that the physicians of 50 years ago were on the right track even though they did not have access to present day scientific

[3] *Ibid.*

equipment. Emil Weiss, M.D., of Chicago, wrote a story for *The Medical Record* for June 4, 1941.[4] In it he described a series of experiments conducted on 22 patients. Every one of these subjects had well known histories of intestinal disorders. Several weeks before the experiments began, daily specimens of urine and feces were collected. Their entire digestive processes were observed and carefully noted. The group of subjects were then divided, and garlic was given to one part of the group while the others took no medication. During the garlic treatment mild diarrhea, headaches and other symptoms of intestinal trouble vanished. We are told that there was a complete change in the intestinal flora (bacteria living in the digestive tract) of those who had taken garlic. Some of these bacteria are very helpful, aiding with the digestion of food, while others are harmful and their presence results in a condition of putrefaction and ill health. It was noted that at the end of the garlic treatments the harmful bacteria were decreasing while the beneficial ones were increasing.

T. D. Yanovich wrote an article describing his experiments with garlic in the *Comptes Rendus de l'Academie des Sciences de l'U.S.S.R.,* 1954, Vol. 48, number 7.[5] He introduced garlic juice directly into the colonies of bacteria and found that all movement of the bacteria ceased within 3 minutes. He also added garlic juice to a culture of bacteria and found that this caused the bacteria to disperse to the edge of the culture. Immobile bacteria began to appear after 2 minutes and all activity had ceased within the short space of ten minutes. It was also found that the freshly prepared juice was much more effective than juice that had been either diluted or preserved for several months.

An old copy of a German medical magazine entitled

[4] *Ibid.*
[5] *Ibid.*

Münchner Medizinische Wochenschrift, Sept. 25, 1925, carried an article written by Professor E. Roos of St. Joseph's Hospital, Freiburg, Germany.[6] In the introduction to this article he states:

> Lack of time and space prevents me from going into more detail on the interesting history of this plant [garlic] as a medical and popular remedy. Its use is age-old. It was used by Hippocrates and Paracelsus and is frequently mentioned in the herbals of the Middle Ages as a remedy. Its range of uses was extremely varied. In recent times, garlic has been highly recommended in France, particularly as a remedy in the case of lung diseases attended by copious and ill-smelling expectoration, as well as a remedy against hypertension.

In his article, Dr. Roos writes mostly of his experiences in treating a variety of intestinal complaints. Some remarkable case histories are given. For example, a laboratory assistant accidently infected herself with a bacteria which causes dysentery. She developed alarming symptoms . . . no appetite, vomiting, diarrhea, followed by bloody stools. She was weak, exhausted and pain-wracked. This woman was given a garlic preparation, two grams, five times a day for six days. Almost at once, the vomiting stopped and she found she could eat again. On the 19th day the illness began to subside, but for quite some time before this, she was able to be out of bed and felt cheerful.

Dr. Roos commented that:

> I could not maintain that the length of time of actual illness was considerably shortened, only that convalescence transpired in a surprisingly rapid man-

[6] J. I. Rodale, *The Encyclopedia for Healthful Living,* Rodale Books, Inc., Emmaus, Pennsylvania, 1960.

ner. To everyone experienced with cases of dysentery the contrast must be extremely surprising between the obviously very severe form of the disease and the extremely light discomfort following introduction of treatment, along with only a mildly exhausted condition.

Here are just a few of the other cases that Dr. Roos mentions:

1. A patient complained that he had suffered from gas, dyspepsia and colitis for 17 years. Occasionally, the diarrhea alternated with spells of constipation. He was given two grams of the garlic preparation two to three times daily. In two and a half months the patient considered himself cured.

2. Two patients, age 36 and 47, suffered from gas, bloating, diarrhea, heart palpitations and headaches. All symptoms were removed after taking garlic for six weeks.

3. A 24-year-old woman suddenly experienced extreme body pains, chills, fever, nausea and diarrhea. She took two grams of garlic three times a day for five days and became completely normal.

4. A 23-year-old student complained of loss of weight, restlessness, excessive gas, and diarrhea. He was returned to normal after taking garlic, with only a brief relapse.

5. A woman patient of 59 suffered from diarrhea for almost nine months. When she first began taking garlic, only a slight improvement was noted, but after six weeks her stools were normal and she was in good health. Examination before garlic treatment was ad-

ministered showed infiltration of harmful bacteria in her stools. When treatment was completed these had vanished.

American Research on Garlic

We know that garlic has been used for centuries in all parts of the world, however it has only been within the past 25 years or so that its use in America is becoming more widespread. Two New York doctors tell of their experiences in using garlic products in an article written in the *New York Physician* for September 1937.[7] Edward H. Kotin, M.D., and David Stein, M.D., review the findings of other researchers on garlic before telling of their own experiences. In presenting this review they mention that it has been found therapeutically useful for the following purposes: It is a harmless yet powerful agent in preventing diptheria, typhus, tuberculosis and pneumonia; it is an expectorant and very useful in all respiratory infections, especially in symptoms of a dry hacking cough, in colds, asthma and bronchitis. Because it stimulates the gastric juices, it is an aid in feeble digestion. It is a wonderful carminative as it relieves dyspepsia, colic and flatulence. It is beneficial to healthful bacteria in the intestines as it stimulates their growth. It kills round and thread worms; therefore it can be classed as an anthelmintic. Diarrhea from infectious diseases such as diptheria, scarlet fever, and tuberculosis respond favorably to garlic therapy. It is a counter-irritant and rubefacient and may be used with advantage in compress form for pleurisy, tuberculosis of the larynx, intercostal neuralgia and catarrhal pneumonia. It is an excellent nerve tonic.

These two doctors then tell of their own experiences in treating patients with garlic. Twelve case histories are given and it is noted that these cases ranged from tuber-

7 Rodale, *The Health Finder*.

culosis to bronchitis, asthma, shortness of breath, constipation, nausea, vomiting, diarrhea, pharyngitis, nervousness, cramps, heartburn, flatulence, chills and fever, chest and abdominal cases. Every single case obtained relief within one month, some within one week. The physicians concluded by saying, ". . . we feel that garlic is an excellent medicament for employment in a diversity of conditions. We believe that the vitamin and mineral factors do much to cause this to be a drug of noteworthy usage."

Treating Colds With Garlic

Dr. J. Klosa experimented with garlic, and reported his findings in an issue of the German magazine entitled *Medical Monthly,* for March 1950.[8] He found that garlic oil had the ability to kill dangerous organisms without endangering the organisms that are so vital to the health of the body. We are told that oil of garlic is composed in part of sulfides, and disulfides, and these unite with virus matter in a certain way which inactivates the virus organism so that their harmful effects are brought to a halt and they are prevented from any further activity. This is accomplished so perfectly, that absolutely no harm is done to the beneficial organisms in the body.

Dr. Klosa experimented with a specially prepared solution of garlic oil and water, which was administered in doses of 10 to 25 drops every 4 hours. The fresh extract of onion juice was also included in the dosage. He reports the results with grippe, sore throat, and rhinitis (clogged and running nose) patients. The fever and catarrhal symptoms of 13 cases of grippe were cut short in every case. Not one of the patients suffered from the usual post-grippe complaints such as swelling of the lymph glands, jaundice, pains in the muscles and joints, chronic

[8] Rodale, *The Encyclopedia for Healthful Living.*

inflammation of the lungs, etc. All patients showed a definite lessening of the required period of convalescence.

In 28 cases of sore throat, the burning and tickling effect abated to a point of disappearance in 24 hours. If caught in its first stages, it was found that further development of sore throat could be stopped completely by administering about 30 drops, or about two doses of the oil of garlic solution.

In 71 cases of clogged and running nose, the oil was taken partly by mouth and partly by being administered directly into the nostrils. In 13 to 20 minutes, the nasal congestion was completely cleared up in all cases and there were no further complications.

Another Medical Opinion on the Value of Garlic in Colds, Etc.

Kristine Nolfi, M.D., refers to the value of garlic in her book *My Experiences With Living Food.*[9] Here are a few excerpts:

> Garlic has a strengthening and laxative effect, lowers too high blood-pressure and raises one which is too low;[10] it also cures indigestion, disinfects the contents of the stomachs of those who lack hydrochloric acid in their gastric juice for this purpose, kills putrefaction bacteria in the large intestine and neutralizes poisons in the organism itself.
>
> If one puts a piece of garlic in his mouth, at the onset of a cold, on both sides between cheek and teeth, the cold will disappear within a few hours or, at most, within a day.
>
> At "Humlegaarden" (Danish health resort) epidemic colds are unknown. Everyone knows that he

[9] Humlegaarden, Humlebaek, Denmark.

[10] Evidence has been shown that garlic is a blood pressure regulator.

must use garlic when a cold begins. Since a cold may develop into pneumonia in the case of weak patients, it is better avoided.

A manufacturer from Bergen in Norway, who has been at "Humlegaarden" several times, was visited one day by a farmer who had a very bad cold. The manufacturer gave him a handful of garlic and told him how to use it. Two days later the farmer telephoned to say that his whole family was well again—their colds had disappeared.

Garlic has also a curative effect on chronic diseases in the upper respiratory organs provided one keeps garlic in his mouth day and night (not while sleeping) renewing the cloves every morning and evening after they have absorbed the poisons. This applies to chronic inflammation of the tonsils, salivary glands and neighboring lymph glands, empyema of the maxillary sinus, severe pharyngitis and laryngitis, bronchitis . . . Garlic makes loose teeth take root again, removes tartar, and has a curative effect on eye catarrh and inflammation of the lacrymal duct, as well as on inflammation of the middle ear. In the latter case, a small clove of garlic may be packed in gauze and placed in the external auditory meatus.

Pimples disappear without leaving a scar if rubbed several times daily with garlic, but this does not prevent the formation of new pimples. Purification of the skin must take place through the blood.

In the desert territories in Finland, where it is difficult to get enough vitamins during the winter, people often make long journeys under unbelievable hardships to get garlic.

During World War II, the Russians discovered that garlic placed on the lip of unclean wounds of soldiers cleaned those wounds in four or five days. Grated garlic placed near the most vicious bacteria will kill them in five minutes.

Laboratory Research on Garlic and Cancer

Some interesting facts were revealed in a research report in *Science*, Vol. 126, Nov. 29, 1957, pg. 1112, that appears to prove that garlic is powerful against tumor-formation.[11]

Austin S. Weisberger and Jack Pensky of Western Reserve University experimented by injecting cancerous cells into mice which produced a rapid cancerous growth and death in 16 days. They obtained the same results even when they treated the cancerous cells with an enzyme they had isolated from garlic. The garlic enzyme by itself had no power to protect against cancer. However, when the cancerous cells were treated not only with the garlic enzyme alone *but also* with an equal amount of the substrate present in garlic, they found that no deaths occurred among the animals for a period of six months, when injected with the treated cells. (The six-month period for the animals is approximately a fourth of a lifetime of a human being.)

The researchers made further experiments by inoculating the mice with virulent cancer cells and then gave them garlic injections. The garlic delayed the development of the malignant tumor and in some cases completely prevented its formation, saving the lives of the mice. In all cases it was absolutely necessary to continue administering the garlic preparation as it was found that the tumors grew rapidly if this was not done.

Garlic and Whooping Cough

The following article by David Reeder, M.D., appeared in *Nature's Path Magazine*.

[11] Rodale, *The Encyclopedia for Health Living.*

Sometime ago at a meeting or convention of physicians in London, a very prominent member gave a talk on whooping cough.

He made the statement, after the lengthy scientific talk about the dangerous character of the disease and the advisability of quarantine, that whooping cough actually caused more deaths among children than any other of the childhood diseases.

He then told them that in the face of all that medical science had been able to do, he had been for several years using a simple home remedy which had been described to him by an old grandmother who was the wise and helpful neighborhood nurse.

She had used it for fifteen years and had never lost a child from whooping cough, and he had used it for five years and had not lost a patient either.

I, personally, have used it and recommended it for more than a dozen years, and have never known of or heard of a child even being made cross-eyed or deaf by the disease when the directions were followed.

Garlic is the remedy, and if it is not already in the home, it is easily procured.

It must be used in the form of a poultice on the bottoms of the feet. This sounds very simple but care should be taken to do the simplest thing right.

Remove the outer shells from the small sections or cloves of the garlic and chop them finely, enough to make a poultice about one-fourth of an inch thick to cover the bottom of each foot, spread it evenly on a piece of soft cloth, then place a thin piece of cloth over the garlic, remembering to grease the bottoms of the feet with lard, vaseline, or similar grease, for if the garlic is placed directly on the feet without the grease, the child cannot stand it as it is apt to blister; now place the prepared poultice on a cloth suitable for binding it on for overnight. It is wise to cover the foot and poultice with an old sock so the poultice will not be kicked off during the night.

Remove it carefully in the morning, as the same poultice may be used several times. After that make a fresh one and proceed as before. You will smell garlic on the patient's breath next morning after the application.

This same treatment will work very satisfactorily in the case of anyone having a hard night cough.

A quiet, comfortable sleep without the usual vomiting of the supper is the usual result of this simple home treatment . . .

The Value of Garlic in Other Disorders

Garlic has been found effective in relieving nicotine poisoning (Dr. Madaus, *idem,* vol. 1, p. 472).

Research conducted by G. Catar, Slovenska University, Bratislava, Czechoslovakia, showed that garlic repels and kills the ticks that carry encephalitis. This is a disease that causes inflammation of the brain in mankind.

Garlic has been scientifically tested in lip and mouth diseases. D. M. Sergaiev and I. D. Leonov, two scientists at the District Oncological Dispensary, Kirovograd, U.S.S.R., have treated 194 cases of such disorders.[12] A paste was made by rubbing garlic in a mortar and then placed on sterile gauze and applied to the affected lip and retained from 8 to 12 hours. Complete healing was reported in over 90 percent of such disorders as leucoplakia (white spots), hyperkeratosis (a horny swelling), and fissures and ulcers of the lip.

Fujiwara, a Japanese scientist, recently discovered that certain substances in garlic increased the body's capacity to assimilate vitamin B_1.

The use of garlic reduced the blood sugar in a case of diabetes (Dr. Madaus, *Lehrbuch der Biologischen Heilmittle,* vol. 1, p. 479).

[12] *Ibid.*

Garlic in India

Herbal medicine is known and used in almost every part of the world, but the systematic study and use of medicinal plants in India can scarcely be equalled anywhere. About two thousand plants are listed in the Ayurvedic, Unani, and Tibbi systems of medicine. The abundance and variety of plants in the regions of India have yielded a great mass of popular herbal remedies through the ages, and these systems provide the most widely used treatment for the people of that vast subcontinent.

Recent efforts have been made to modernize these great systems, and though the plants are still locally used in crude form, the advancement of pharmaceutical researches is resulting in the exploitation of many of the herbs. As the active principles of the plants are being scientifically isolated in pure forms, the manufacture of these "secret" remedies is now a growing commercial industry. Modern day pharmacological, chemical, microbiological, clinical and other procedures are being used.

In his book, *Medicinal Plants of India and Pakistan*,[13] the author describes the plants used for drugs and remedies according to the Ayurvedic, Unani, Tibbi systems and those mentioned in American and British pharmacopoeias. Among these is garlic, and he relates its value and use as follows:

Uses: Garlic resembles squill (Urginea maritima) in its medicinal properties; it is given in fevers, coughs, flatulence, disorders of the nervous system, agues, dropsical affections, pulmonary phthisis, whooping cough, . . . and dilated bronchi. It has diuretic and emmenagogic properties as well. A decoction of garlic

[13] J. F. Dastur, F.N.I. (D. B. Taraporevala Sons & Co. Private Ltd., Bombay, India), 1962, 2nd Ed.

made with milk and water is given in small doses in hysteria, flatulence, sciatica, etc. Garlic in the form of a syrup is a valuable remedy for asthma, hoarseness and disorders of the chest and lungs. As an anthelmintic, the juice of garlic is given in doses of 10 to 30 drops; garlic syrup is given in doses of a drachm.

Externally, garlic is used as a rubefacient, vesicant and disinfectant. It is applied to indolent tumors, ulcerated surfaces and wounds; a poultice of the bulb is used for scrofulous sores and ringworm. A clove of garlic is introduced in the ear passage for relief of earache. As a rubefacient, garlic is locally used in sciatica, paralysis and neuralgic pains. A garlic poultice is applied on the abdominal and pubic regions in retention of urine due to atony of the bladder. Raw garlic juice is inhaled in whooping cough and pulmonary tuberculosis. The oil in which garlic has been fried is a useful liniment for rheumatic pains, nervous diseases . . .

The oil extracted from the seeds is given for checking cold fits of intermittent fevers. As a liniment, it is used for paralytic and rheumatic affections.

IV

the wonder remedy of bygone days

. . . and the vine do yield their strength.
—Joel 2:22.

SARSAPARILLA *(Smilax officinalis)* is the dried root of the
smilax, a genus of climbing or trailing vines or shrubs native to tropical America. The name is derived from two
Spanish words, *sarza* and *parilla,* meaning a small, thorny
vine. The plant grows only in moist places and develops
long, slender roots.

There are several varieties of the sarsaparilla of commerce, a few of which are mentioned as follows: Mexi-
can, Vera Cruz, Tampico or *grey* sarsaparilla, Honduras
or *brown* sarsaparilla, Jamaica, Costa Rica, Central
American or *red* sarsaparilla, Guayaquil sarsaparilla
found in the valleys and western slopes of the Andes, and
Ecuadorian sarsaparilla which has been on the American
market since 1935. The root (rhizome) of *Smilax china*
is native to China and Japan, and has been used under
the name of *China Root* for similar purposes with the official sarsaparilla.

Authorities state that care must be taken in selecting
the sarsaparilla of commerce as it may be found to be

59

nearly or entirely inert due to age or because it was obtained from an inferior species. We are told that a practical criterion in determining good sarsaparilla is in the taste. If, after having chewed a piece of the root for a short time, a decidedly acrid impression is left in the mouth, the sarsaparilla may be considered of good quality; if not, it is probably inert.

Early Medical Use of Sarsaparilla

Sarsaparilla was the wonder remedy of bygone days, and was considered a necessity by many people for good health. Writings on the virtues of the plant could be found in almanacs and newspapers, while old time drug stores carried a wide variety of sarsaparilla preparations.

Few medicines have undergone greater changes of reputation. Sarsaparilla was introduced into Europe around the middle of the 16th century as a remedy for venereal disease, for which purposes it had been lauded in the early Spanish settlements of the West Indies. It soon fell into disuse until revived by Sir William Fordyce in 1757. For more than 100 years it continued to be regarded valuable as an alternative, not only in syphilis but in chronic rheumatism, scrofula, and various skin diseases. During the latter part of the 19th century, the medicinal use of sarsaparilla was considered only the survival of ignorant superstition, and would have disappeared completely from medical attention had it not been that the plant contained valuable properties as a vehicle of the compound syrup. However, after an extensive review of more recent evidence, Perutz (Handb. d Haut-und Geschlechteskrank, 1928) arrived at the conclusion that sarsaparilla does have some value in the treatment of syphilis, probably by stimulating the body's defensive mechanism.

Sarsaparilla and Psoriasis [1]

A report of the successful use of a water extract of sarsaparilla in the treatment of psoriasis was given by Philippsohn (Derm. Wchnschr., 1931, 93, 1220). He advised his patients to put 15 gm. of sarsaparilla in 1000 ml. of tepid water and allow the mixture to stand over night. On the following morning they were instructed to boil the mixture for 20 minutes and immediately drink half of the infusion while it was still hot, and take the remainder during the day. This practice was to be repeated daily. We are told that a week later "decreased desquamation" (peeling of the skin) took place. After its complete disappearance, there was a marked smooth "red macule" (blemish) which eventually faded. One patient with a previously stubborn case of psoriasis followed the treatment daily for 20 years without a single relapse at any time.

Tablets containing sarsaparilla were used with good results in the treatment of psoriasis by Grutz and Bürger (Klin. Wchnschr., 1933, 12, 373) and Ritter (Deutsche med. Wchnschr., 1936, 62, 1629).

Sas-par (Bischoff) tablets made from substances found in Honduras sarsaparilla were administered to 75 patients with psoriasis by Thurmon (New Eng. J. Med., 1942, 227, 128). A decided beneficial effect was noted in 62 percent of the cases.

Further Research on Sarsaparilla [2]

A search for hormones in plant substances was under-

[1] The Dispensatory of the United States of America, 25th Edition (Osol-Farrar), J. B. Lippincott Company, Philadelphia, 1955.

[2] Dr. Leon De Seblo, *Sickness and Senility Are Unnecessary*, Health Research, Molelumne Hill, California.

taken several years ago by two American research men, Professor Russell E. Marker and Dr. Aval Rohrmon of Pennsylvania State College. Hundreds of plants were tested in their search for hormones or what may be termed pro-hormones. Repeatedly they thought they had discovered a hormone in a plant only to be disappointed in the end. It was not until 1939 that they began to experiment with an extract of the roots of sarsaparilla. This time they were successful and in the same year they announced that sarsaparilla root contained hormones.

The first hormone found by the two research scientists was the male hormone, testosterone. Their announcement of this fact was scarcely noticed by the medical world. It was not until an issue of the *New York Times,* August 11, 1946, carried the story of a discovery in Mexico of the male hormone in sarsaparilla that sufficient notice was given to the matter. Progesterone and cortin are two other hormones that have been extracted from the root of the plant.

It appears that the discoveries in America and Mexico were made independently of each other. Dr. Eric Solmo, a Hungarian scientist, had lived in Mexico for a number of years and was curious about a "remedy" used by the Indians as a cure for physical debility, weakness, and sexual impotence. He decided to investigate the merits of this remedy, and made exhaustive tests with sarsaparilla root. His findings were the same as those of Rohrman and Marker. Dr. Solmo conducted thousands of laboratory tests on animals and men, and proved beyond a doubt that sarsaparilla hormones do benefit their users.

Testosterone and Impotence [8]

The inability of a man to exercise his normal sex function is called impotence. Medical men say that this weak-

[8] *Ibid.*

ness often alters a man's personality and distorts his entire outlook on life. He may develop an inferiority complex as he begins to think of himself as only half a man. Scientists tell us that impotence is generally due to the inability of the testicles to supply the body with a normal supply of the male hormone.

Various experiments have shown that the administration of testosterone tends to restore sexual power, mental alertness and physical strength to men who are entering the aging process of physical decline. In a sense, testosterone prolongs youth and prevents premature aging. It was also noted that even in short duration experiments, sallow dry skin, usually a mark of old age, became healthy and clear, and mental and physical powers were decidedly increased. However, as in the case of diabetics who must continue taking insulin shots, the beneficial effects of the male hormone are in evidence only so long as the hormone is taken. Mexico and South American countries now manufacture testosterone tablets made from sarsaparilla root.

Testosterone and Angina Pectoris [4]

Experiments have been made with the use of testosterone in cases of angina pectoris. Scientists explain that this heart ailment results from the fact that the heart muscle is starved for oxygen, and consequently becomes painfully cramped. Results obtained by the use of testosterone offer hope in the future for this type of heart patient.

During his service as Assistant Professor of Internal Medicine at Harvard University, Dr. Samuel W. Levine carefully examined the reports of results obtained through the administration of testosterone to people suffering from diseases of the blood vessels of the legs and feet. He asked himself this question: "If testosterone conditions

[4] Ibid.

damaged blood vessels so that more blood can reach the feet and legs, why then cannot that same testosterone condition the coronary arteries so that more blood can reach the heart muscles, thereby alleviating the spasms of angina pectoris?"

Dr. Levine experimented and observed that one-fourth of his patients showed decided improvement at the end of four weeks' treatment. These experiments were, of course, too short in duration to definitely prove the value of testosterone with respect to this ailment. At that time, however, an extract of the male hormone could be obtained only from animals, and the high cost necessitated the discontinuance of his experiments.

At a later time, similar tests were made by Dr. M. A. Lesser, and the results were found to be the same. Real improvement was noted in all his patients in a short time. They were able to tolerate more physical exertion than before taking the testosterone treatment, and were free of the usual resulting heart spasms. The paroxysms were also less severe and were less frequent.

Other medical colleges and physicians have since tested the male hormone in the treatment of angina pectoris. All agreed that testosterone did minimize the painful paroxysms of angina pectoris, and may possibly abolish them completely. However, the treatment must be indefinitely continued if the favorable effects are to be maintained.

Testosterone and Baldness

An interesting article appeared in the *San Francisco News Call Bulletin*, Dec. 16, 1964.[5] In it, Dr. Christopher M. Papa, a resident in dermatology of the University of Pennsylvania Hospital, revealed that he had been able to

[5] Associated Press, as reported in the *News Call Bulletin*, San Francisco.

grow hair on the heads of 21 bald men, and produced photographs as well as other proof to back up his claim.

It appears that Dr. Papa's discovery came about by accident as it was a "by-product of other research." He confesses that "we didn't set out to grow hair," and adds, "but we found that we were doing it as we rubbed the hormone drug *testosterone* on the skin under the arm pits." Subsequently the hormone was tried on the head and it was found that the hair grew. Dr. Papa points out that it took many months, "but it grew." In one case, it was a year before any noticeable effects were observed. He mentions that he is very happy to have been able to make a break-through in hair-growing research, and stresses the fact that up until the present time baldness was considered hopeless. Now he is convinced that it isn't. He says: "Man can grow hair, which makes the process of losing hair reversible."

Dr. Papa insists that his discovery is still in the experimental stage and that much more study must be made. He carefully points out that, "I'm not in private practice," and adds that, "I wouldn't dare advise you, or anyone else, to use this testosterone, which happens to be an old-time drug which can be obtained only by prescription. It should be used only on the advice of a physician."

Dr. Papa, though sympathetic about the baldness problem, was not interested in following through with further research on this himself.

Progesterone [6]

Progesterone is another of the valuable hormones found in sarsaparilla. This is the hormone that medical men tell us is normally produced by the ovaries in the female. It is said to be necessary for the development of the mammary and genital organs, and essential for reproduc-

[6] De Seblo.

tion. We are further informed that progesterone is found in the corpus luteum, a yellow mass within the ovary. The corpus luteum aids the condition of the womb in making preparation for pregnancy, and also tends to prevent miscarriage. Progesterone is said to quiet the muscles of the womb and ease the spasmodic pains which sometimes follow childbirth.

Cortin [7]

Researchers have found that sarsaparilla also contains cortin, one of the hormones secreted by the adrenal glands. According to medical science, the body dies almost immediately if the supply of this vital hormone is completely cut off. On the other hand, if the adrenal glands secrete only a small or insufficient amount of cortin, the individual becomes easy prey to infectious diseases and also develops nervous depression and general weakness.

The Future of Sarsaparilla

The presence of hormones and other substances scientifically identified in sarsaparilla has brought this cast-off herb once again into prominence. Science has now established a new reputation for sarsaparilla which may lead us to believe that the plant will find a lasting place among the materia medica of modern man.

[7] *Ibid.*

V

a magic herb of proven value

And I will raise up for them a plant of renown.
—Ezk. 34:29.

COMFREY (*Symphytum officinale*) is a native of Europe, but is naturalized in the United States, growing on low grounds and moist places. The root is spindle-shaped, branched, and penetrates deeply into the earth. The plant was used by the early herbalists in the treatment of a variety of ailments, but it was not until centuries later that its value was realized by men of science. In his book, *Narrative of an Investigation Concerning an Ancient Medicinal Remedy and Its Modern Utilities,*[1] Charles J. Macalister, M.D., of England, relates how he became acquainted with the healing power of comfrey and his subsequent discoveries regarding it.

An Accidental Discovery

Dr. Macalister tells us that between the years 1910-

[1] Lee Foundation For Nutritional Research (Milwaukee, Wisc.), 1962.

1911, he was looking for an important paper that he had had published in the *Lancet* in 1896. While searching through this old issue of the *Lancet,* he came across an interesting article entitled, "Some Surprises and Mistakes," by Professor William Thompson, President of the Royal College of Surgeons in Ireland. This article cited the case of a man, "who was suffering from a tumour involving the nose and antrum, which on being removed, was declared to be a round-celled sarcoma by Dr. O'Sullivan, Professor of Pathology in Trinity College, Dublin." We are told that the growth, however, reappeared, and the patient then consulted Sir Felix Simon who advised that the jaw be removed. It was agreed and the operation performed. A month later the growth had once again returned and was now bulging through the incision, almost closing the right eye. As further operation was impossible the man was sent home.

The article stated that three months later the patient called on Professor Thompson who declared that he had never seen the man looking better. There was no longer a trace of the tumour either on his face or in his mouth. The patient informed the astonished Professor that he had applied poultices of comfrey to the affected parts and that the tumour had gradually disappeared. In his article, Professor Thompson said, "I am as satisfied as can be that the growth was malignant and of a bad type—I know nothing of the effects of comfrey root but I do not believe that it could remove a sarcomatous tumour."

Dr. Macalister remarks that he has known of cases where malignant growths had spontaneously disappeared and that the case just cited may have been one also; however, he was open-minded enough to entertain the possibility that "comfrey might contain some substance capable of controlling or stabilizing cell-growth, and it naturally led to an investigation of the literature of comfrey and to experiments being made with it clinically." Dr. Macalister tells us that prior to reading the article he had never heard of comfrey and that nothing of its properties were taught in the materia medica classes that he had attended as a student.

Use of the "Magic" Herb in Bygone Days

In searching through old herbals, he did, however, find that it was held as an important remedy in bygone days. From these antiquated books he read such things as the following references to comfrey. (The old-time spelling is preserved where found).

From Turner's *Herball* (1568):

> Of Comfrey Symphytum. The rootes are good if they be broken and dronken for them that spitte blood, and are bursten. The same, layd to, are good to glewe together freshe woundes. They are also good to be layd to inflammation, and specially of the fundament, with the leaves of groundsell.

Parkinson's *Theatrum Botanicum* (1640) states:

> The rootes of Comfrey, taken fresh, beaten small, spread upon leather, and laid upon any place troubled with the gout, doe presently give ease of the paines; and applyed in the same manner, giveth ease to pained joynts, and profiteth very much for running and moist ulcers, gangrenes, mortifications, and the like.

An Amazing Discovery

After Dr. Macalister became acquainted with the history of the plant and the various ways in which it had been employed as a remedy in the past, he decided to put the plant to use in medical practice. The results he achieved through this and the subsequent chemical analysis proved that comfrey contained a valuable healing agent. This healing agent is called *allantoin,* a cell proliferant, found in the leaves and roots of comfrey.

Dr. Macalister cites some interesting case histories. In referring to gastric and other internal ulcerations, he says:

A woman, aged 47, was admitted to my ward in an extremely debilitated condition in consequence of a severe attack of haematemesis. For many weeks previously she had suffered from pain after food, and had vomited persistently for a fortnight prior to her admission. Even water caused pain and was immediately rejected. There had been melaena for some time prior to the attack of haematemesis for which she was immediately admitted. For 12 months she had been conscious of pain on pressure over the abdomen, and had noticed a lump in the epigastrium and extending into the right hypochondrium. This woman was so feeble that the ward sister (nurse) said that she thought it was a pity that a patient so ill and advanced in disease should be sent into the hospital. I felt disposed to agree with this opinion, because on examining her abdomen I found a tumour just beneath the ribs on the right side. It was rounded, irregular, and intensely painful, and my feeling at the time was that she had a carcinoma involving the stomach . . . When the irritability of the stomach subsided she was given the mucilaginous infusion of Comfrey root reinforced with some of the saturated solution of allantoin. In addition to the improvement which took place in her stomach symptoms, in the course of a month the abdominal tumour disappeared, an area remaining, however, which was extremely painful on pressure; but in time this also disappeared, and what I had taken to be a malignant growth had vanished.

We are told of another astonishing case which was transferred to the care of Dr. Macalister. The patient was a 48-year-old woman:

There was a large ulcer on the dorsum of the foot
and another practically continuous with it, over the
lower third of the leg. The bases were in places
sloughy and even gangrenous looking, and there was
a purulent discharge. She was sent to Dr. Crawford,
I understood, for his opinion as to whether the leg
should be amputated. The ulcer measured five in. by
four in., and had been in existence for five years.
Allantoin dressings were commenced on July 25. A
week later the surface had cleaned and presented
healthy granulations, and a rapid growth of epithelium
was taking place from all the margins. On August 12
it was manifestly healing, and on August 17, i.e., in
23 days, this huge ulcer was reduced to the size of a
pin's head. The scar was healthy and sound. The
patient was kept in bed for a fortnight, and after her
discharge it remained sound and well.

Results Obtained by Other Physicians

Dr. Macalister also mentions some of the results obtained by other physicians. A patient having a very deep
burn of the eyeball and lids, due to contact with molten
copper, was treated by an ophthalmic surgeon who employed allantoin dressings. The surgeon reported that "the
disappearance of the chemosis, the firm healing of the
deeper layers and the formation of new tissue have been
most marked and have even astonished the nurses who
know nothing about the stuff."

Dr. Charles Searle of Cambridge tells of a patient, a
man 83 years of age, whom he first saw on Oct. 23,
1911. The man suffered from swelling of the legs and
shortness of breath. We are told that for some months his
condition was grave as he had marked arteriosclerosis,
feeble pulse, low temperature and a "loud aortic systolic
murmur." There was evidence of blood, albumin, and
casts in the urine, but no sugar. Dr. Searle reported:

During December, 1911, a fungating ulcer appeared on the dorsum of the left foot. It rapidly spread, and eventually exposed the metatarsal bones. In January, 1912, the patient's condition appeared to be hopeless, he became at times delirious, and was removed home to die. He was then treated with four-hourly fomentations made with decoction of Comfrey root. The ulcer immediately began to fill up rapidly and was practically healed by the end of April, and the patient's condition made corresponding improvement.

In referring to the remarkable work cited in his book, Dr. Macalister says:

Much of the earlier work was carried out many years ago and some of it was published in the *British Medical Journal*. New matter is included in this record which has been written by way of opening the door for further investigations by those who may feel interested enough to avail themselves of clinical opportunities which, in my retirement, I do not possess. (1936)

A dedicated and open-minded physician of more recent years who became "interested enough" in the value of comfrey is H. E. Kirschner, M.D. In his book, *Nature's Healing Grasses*,[2] he devotes four chapters to the subject of comfrey alone. He tells us that his interest in the plant started in the latter part of 1956 when he set out a large bed of comfrey in his garden. It is obvious from Dr. Kirschner's writings on the subject that his experience with the medicinal use of comfrey substantiates many of the claims made by the old-time herbalists, as well as the findings of Dr. Macalister.

[2] H. C. White Publications, Yucaipa, Calif., 1960.

Two Interesting Cases

Recently [says Dr. Kirschner] a most interesting case came under my observation. A middle-aged woman came to me with a large . . . ulcer below the eye and close to the nose. I prescribed a comfrey poultice, and the "Green Drink", containing comfrey leaves. Soon after the application of the comfrey leaf poultice, the painful swelling subsided, and rapid improvement was noted. Only a few months after the initial treatment there was a complete healing over of the infected area . . .

Another interesting case has just come to my attention. The patient is a woman 86 years of age who lives with her husband in a Sanitarium in nearby Azusa. Some months ago she was afflicted with a troublesome growth on the right side of her nose. This ugly, red, nipple-shaped growth was treated by her doctor in the regular orthodox manner. But unfortunately this curative measure was of short duration, and very soon the growth was back again . . .

Her son became deeply concerned over his mother's condition, and having read my articles about the miracle-working properties of comfrey in *Let's Live Magazine*, he suggested that perhaps an old-fashioned comfrey-root poultice might relieve this ugly, fast growing "wart." She and her husband agreed to try this simple remedy, and the following day her son mailed a little bottle of dried comfrey root powder to his mother.

Small poultices were immediately applied to her nose during the daytime and a large poultice was worn at night. Almost immediately the inflamed condition subsided, and the nasty growth began to recede. The recession was slow but gradual, and in less than 60 days the once ugly "wart" had completely disappeared. Today even close examination fails to show a trace of this once distressing growth, and there are no tell-tale scars.

Dr. Kirschner also tells us of a report he received from New Zealand dealing with the use of comfrey. He states that, "This story from 'down under' confirms all that I have written about this miracle-working plant, and should bring renewed hope to those of my readers who are afflicted with the distressing symptoms of asthma." He quotes the report as follows:

> A farmer friend casually nibbled a comfrey leaf in the front yard of Mrs. D. H. Johnson, of Cambridge, New Zealand. As a result she is now overwhelmed with requests for the leaf. Already it has helped hundreds of sufferers with a wide range of complaints.
>
> This friend had suffered from asthma for thirty years. His first night of unbroken sleep followed. Trying to trace the reason for this unusual experience, he thought back over his action of the previous day. He decided it must be the comfrey leaf he had eaten and sent for more. Now he eats some every day and has not suffered from asthma since. Mrs. Johnson's own son also suffered from asthma. He followed the same routine and was similarly relieved.

We are told that supplies of comfrey leaves are shipped all over New Zealand today from the Johnson farm. Letters come to Mrs. Johnson almost daily from people suffering from such things as rheumatic complaints, digestive disorders, eczema and other skin troubles, boils and varicose ulcers, as well as asthma. All these people claim that they eat better, sleep better and feel "much fitter, following a 'course' of comfrey leaves."

How to Use Comfrey

Dr. Kirschner says that he gets many letters from people asking how they should use comfrey. In cases of obstinate ulcers, burns, open wounds, or inflammation caused by insect bites, he says that a poultice may be prepared by putting the comfrey leaves through a juicer. He further explains, however, that:

> —as the comfrey leaves contain little juice, but a thick mucilaginous substance, like okra, the macerated leaves are gathered from the "basket" of the juicer following the operation, and not the spout, the mass of triturated comfrey leaves can then be spread on a cloth and applied to the infected area.

A meat grinder or hand grater is suggested if a centrifugal electric juicer is not available, or the leaves may be placed on a board using a hammer to macerate them. Dr. Kirschner suggests from 10 to 12 medium-size leaves be used when making a large poultice as just mentioned. Powdered comfrey root dampened with enough water to form a sticky mucilaginous mass, then spread on a cloth and placed on the infected area, is another method he suggests for making a poultice.

In preparing comfrey tea, Dr. Kirschner prefers to use four small, fresh leaves, cutting them up and steeping them as he would ordinary tea. He adds that the dried leaves (desiccated) are a good substitute for the fresh ones and a heaping tablespoonful should be used in preparing the tea.

For preparing the fresh roots of comfrey, he cites the directions given in *Potter's Cyclopaedia of Botanical Drugs and Preparations:* "One-half to one ounce of the crushed root is boiled in one quart of water. The dose is a wineglassful."

With regard to whether the root or leaves of the comfrey plant is the best to use, Dr. Kirschner explains that:

> Some authorities believe that the roots of the comfrey plant are even more potent than the leaves. However, as stated above, both the *leaves* and the *roots* contain the priceless *allantoin,* and, therefore,

we believe *both* can be used effectively as a poultice, or can be taken internally as an additive to food or drink. In fact, long experience has proved this to be so.

The Value of Comfrey Cited by a Swiss Doctor

Dr. Kirschner draws the reader's attention to an informative book, *The Nature Doctor,*[3] written by his friend Dr. Alfred Vogel of Switzerland. It appears that Dr. Vogel also considers comfrey to be a valuable healing agent. Dr. Kirschner quotes him as follows:

> The comfrey plant grows, for the most part unnoticed, near farmyards. Even in ancient times, it has been used to heal wounds, broken bones and especially leg fractures. Considering its value in these cases alone, it would deserve more attention than it usually receives. It encourages the healing process and speeds up the formation of new bone cells which is probably due to the fact that it contains from .08 to 1 per cent of *allantoin*. This is known to promote granulation and the formation of epithelial cells. Cholin is another constituent of the comfrey plant, while other important elements may also be present, although these are, as yet, unknown . . .
>
> Comfrey tincture is an excellent remedy for an injured periosteum, i.e., the outer covering of the bones, and it also has been successfully used for suppurating ulcers, wounds which refuse to heal, and leg ulcers. There is hardly a better remedy to be found for the external treatment of gout.

As Dr. Vogel points out, it was the practice even in ancient times to use comfrey as an accessory remedy for broken bones. It is this value attributed to the herb that has given it the synonym of *knitbone*. Recently, a British researcher, Lawrence D. Hills stated:

[3] Bioforce-Verlag, Teufen (AR), Switzerland, 1959.

We know now what the bone-knitting and healing virtues of comfrey are, because both root and foliage contain *allantoin*, a nitrogenous crystalline substance, which is a cell proliferant, that is, it increases the speed at which nature can heal a wound, internal irritation, or broken bone.

VI

one of man's oldest herbal remedies

A bundle of myrrh is my well-beloved unto me.
—S.S. 1:13.

MYRRH (*Balsamodendron myrrha*) is a shrub or tree native to Abyssinia and other countries bordering upon the Red Sea. It is quite low and branchy, with a whitish-grey bark, and bears fruit about the size of a pea. The juice flows naturally from the bark, forming soft reddish-brown drops or tears which gradually harden and form the medicinal *gum myrrh*. These drops vary in size from that of a small grain to as large as that of an egg. They powder readily, giving off a pleasant balsamic fragrance, and the taste, though bitter, is not unpleasant. The best quality of gum myrrh which is gathered for the market is known as *herabol myrrh*.

A Romantic History

Myrrh is one of man's oldest favorites among the botanicals and its history is a romantic one, filled with legend and lore. Through countless centuries, the little lumps of gum-resin harvested from the myrrh trees played an important role in the trade and commerce of the ancient world of the East.

In the first book of the Old Testament we read: *and, behold, a company of Ish-mee-lites came from Gilead with their camels bearing spicery and balm and myrrh, going to carry it down to Egypt.—Gen. 37:25.* It is significant that this caravan was bound for Egypt, for myrrh was in great demand by the ancient Egyptians who esteemed it highly as one of the chief ingredients in the process of embalming. The art and practice of mummification dates from about 4000 B.C. through 700 A.D. An estimated 750,000,000 bodies, the majority of which were human, while some were those of sacred animals, were embalmed during this period. It was believed by the Egyptians that the soul of the dead who departed from his life in good grace, would eventually return to reclaim the body and enjoy an everlasting physical existence. Thus it was essential that the bodies of the dead be well-preserved during the waiting period which was supposed to cover from 3000 to 10,000 years. It was assumed that during this time, the soul was performing a sort of probationary pilgrimage in the mysterious unknown.

The price of the higher class embalming ranged from approximately $500 to $4500 for each corpse, depending upon the value of the various perfumes, ointments, spices, chemicals, etc., that were employed. During this process all internal organs were removed except the heart and kidneys. The body was then washed and shaved and all of the necessary spices applied. Powerful drugs were used in effecting passage into the various cavities of the skull and different parts of the body. In some instances the nails were gilded, and the fingers and toes encased in costly enclosures of gold. The face was given considerable care and was treated with a coat of fine plaster and expensive chemicals. Once this treatment was completed, the bodies were carefully wrapped in the finest Indian muslin and placed in mummy cases.

The poorer classes, every bit as concerned with their own physical immortality as were the rich, turned to myrrh, the more reasonable preservative, to assure themselves of an everlasting visible existence. The bodies of the poor were washed with myrrh and salted for 70 days. When this was completed, they were wrapped in coarse cloth and placed in catacombs.

How the Ancients Used Myrrh

The ancient Hebrews regarded myrrh as one of the earth's most precious and versatile products, for as a medicine it healed their bodies, as an incense it lifted their spirits and as a perfume it pleased their hearts. Ample evidence of their high regard for myrrh is noted throughout the glorious Song of Solomon. One of its most important uses was as an ingredient in the holy oils with which they anointed the Tabernacle, the Ark, the altar and the sacred vessels. The Book of Esther relates that six of the 12 months devoted to the purification of women were accomplished with oil of myrrh. Unquestionably, the principle behind this purification was spiritual, but it is an interesting possibility that oil of myrrh may have been chosen because of its beneficial effects on the body as well. In many countries, even at the present time, myrrh is used in herbal liniments as a treatment for rheumatism. Ancient Chinese herbalists taught that women are very prone to rheumatic illnesses, due to the monthly loss of blood and the rigors of childbearing. Therefore it is very likely that the Hebrew women were benefited in health by the anointment with oil of myrrh.

Myrrh was also used by the ancient Greeks and is celebrated in their classical mythology. According to one story, a woman named Myrrha gave birth to Adonis, a legendary youth of great beauty. Later, Myrrha was turned into a myrrh tree.

The ancient Persian aristocracy whose private gardens and orchards were masterpieces of horticulture, cultivated myrrh trees for their own use. Of the Three Wise Men, believed to be members of the priestly caste of Persia, one considered myrrh to be of such exceptional value that it was offered by him as a gift to the Infant Jesus, the Highest of Kings.

The chief markets for the spices and botanicals shifted with the rise and fall of the old civilizations. The cities of Alexandria, Cairo, Constantinople, Baghdad, each in its turn became a center for this trade which was a source of fabulous wealth for the merchants. Eventually, with the discovery of the Cape of Good Hope by Bartholomew Diaz in 1486, the Western world became an active participant in this ancient trade, and gradually these products became known the world over. Thus from the cradle of civilization to modern times, myrrh has been on hand to comfort mankind in a variety of ways.

Modern Medical Use of Myrrh

One of the best descriptions of the medicinal uses of myrrh is given by R. Swinburne Clymer, M.D.: [1]

> . . . In whatever form it is used Myrrh will be found to be a powerful antiseptic having for thousands of years been used for preservative purposes, and also as medicine. It is generally administered as a tincture in water or syrup, although the powder may be given to equally good advantage. Two grains of the powdered Myrrh may be considered an average dose, best given combined with other indicated agents.

[1] *The Medicines of Nature,* The Humanitarian Society, Reg., Quakertown, Penna., 1960.

A small teaspoon each of powdered Myrrh and
Golden Seal to a pint of boiling water and a little
ginger added will be found useful to weak stomachs
where the food is prone to ferment. Dose: a teaspoonful every two hours.

Outwardly applied, Myrrh is invaluable for foul
ulcers, bedsores, . . . best mixed with powdered char-
coal. Powdered Myrrh with *Hydrastis* (Golden Seal)
may be sprinkled into indolent sores . . . Powdered
Myrrh is a superior tooth-powder, especially where
the gums are tender and bleeding.

The compound tincture of Myrrh, known as No. 6,
is a powerful stimulant and antiseptic . . . Internally,
a few drops in a glass of water will prove a powerful
stimulant in shock, collapse, prostration and profound
congestion.

No. 6 may be quickly and readily made thus:

Tinct. Myrrh 2 oz.

Tinct. *Capsicum* ½ oz.

Four to eight drops in plenty of water. To make it
more potent, add four ounces of Tincture *Echinacea*.
Dose: ten to fifteen drops in plenty of water.

Myrrh is an active tonic, a stimulant, and is possessed of highly antiseptic properties.

Myrrh has been successfully employed in chronic
diarrhea, and in diseases of the lungs and chest,
attended by a free expectoration and general debility.
It is also well adapted to female complaints, when
unattended by fever.

Applied to fresh wounds, the tincture of Myrrh
excites healing action and lessens the liability to the
occurrence of unhealthy inflammation. It is equally
useful in old sores, ulcerated sore mouth, and ulcerated sore throat, . . . aphthous sore mouth, spongy
gums, and sore nipples.

After a vapor bath, when the patient is rubbed dry,
washing the surface with partly diluted tincture of
Myrrh affords a means of protection against cold,
and strengthens and improves the condition of the
skin. This practice is useful especially in cases where

the skin is relaxed and the patient feeble, as in chronic bronchitis, chronic pleurisy, asthma, chronic rheumatism, chronic diarrhea, marasmus, and in every other form of disease attended by general debility.

In deeply seated colds attended by a free expectoration of a thick yellowish secretion, the use of No. 6, will be found highly beneficial.

An external application of No. 6, *i.e.*, compound tincture Myrrh and *Capsicum*, has been found useful in rheumatism, neuralgia and like ailments.

The compound tincture may be applied to great advantage in sprains, bruises, fresh cuts, indolent ulcers, . . . and as a preventative to mortification both internally and externally.

The Dispensatory of the United States of America [2] (page 877) 25th edition, lists the value of tincture of Myrrh as follows:

Uses.—Myrrh tincture is used as a local application to stimulate spongy gums, aphthous sore mouth, and ulcerations of the throat; diluted, it is employed as a mouth wash in stomatitis and other affections. Internally it has been used as a carminative.

[2] Osol-Farrar, J. B. Lippincott Co., Philadelphia, 1955.

VII

the magic of seeds

*. . . and give us seed, that we may live, and not
die, that the land be not desolate.—Gen. 47:19.*

PLANT SEEDS SUPPLY man with an abundance of foods.
From the first settlement in America, a steady growing
demand arose for seeds of fruits, vegetables and farm
grains. Originally it was customary for farmers as well as
others to preserve their own seed supplies obtained from
their own production. However, the growth of the country and the development of cities soon caused such an increasing demand for seeds that it resulted in the establish-
ment of seed farms. Seed production became the principal
object of these farms whose purpose it was to meet the
demand of those producing materials for the city markets.
The first seed farm was established near Philadelphia by
David Landreth in 1784. At present there are hundreds
of farms in the United States devoted entirely to seed production.

Further Uses of Seeds

From the distant past to the present, pungent and aromatic seeds have been employed for many purposes, most generally as flavoring in cookery. Over 300 years ago Parkinson wrote, "Caraway is much used to be put among baked fruit, or into bread, cakes, etc., to give them relish." Fenugreek seeds are used as a condiment in Egypt, and in curries in India. The people of India also make a gruel of the seeds with sugar and milk. In Mexico, cumin seeds are highly valued as an ingredient in chili powders, while the flavor of coriander seeds is a favorite among many people of South America who use it in almost all their dishes.

Fennel was popular with the early Romans who munched the stalks, and crowned their warriors with garlands of the leaves. The flavorful seeds were ground and crushed for use in masking the taste of unpleasant medicines. Fennel is widely used today in cookery, and also to flavor absinthe and others liqueurs.

Though not generally realized, the use of seeds as a domestic remedy is still employed in many parts of the world today. Orientals enjoy chewing cardamon seeds to sweeten their breath and for the relief of acid stomach. Anise is valued as a diuretic, carminative and pectoral; barley as a strengthening aid in convalescence; caraway for upset stomach and gas; celery for rheumatism. Burdock seed teas are believed to purify the blood and thereby eliminate or prevent sties and boils.

Scientific Research on Seeds

The *American Mercury,* February 1960, carried an article entitled "Seeds That Heal," by Charles H. Coleman. The article states that men of science have been discovering and extracting substances in seeds which may prove valuable as ingredients in many "modern" medicines.

The article mentions that research scientists Bianco Magno and Paolo Rovesti of the Institute for Research on Vegetable Derivatives at Milan, Italy, have found that seeds can be intriguing from a scientific viewpoint. These two scientists take a pile of shelled corn, to which they add water. The grains begin to sprout (without dirt, they cannot grow), and after they have germinated, which usually takes about 10 days, the scientists make their extractions. An enormous amount of pressure is applied through the use of a special press, which squeezes out every drop of the juice. All that remains of the seed itself is a dry pomace.

We are told that many different vitamins, oils, and other substances are contained in corn juice and from the juices of other seeds as well. Dermatological tests have indicated that these juices stimulate and nourish the skin. Consequently, Magno and Rovesti have made up a "special cosmetic from the juices, the pomace, an antibiotic and an antioxidant."

Vitamins Found in Seeds

According to the article, Rovesti and Magno subject a variety of germinated seeds to the process of extraction. They have found that lupine juice contains vitamin A, the vitamin which science tells us is necessary for the health of the eyes and skin; wheat juice, vitamin E believed by some authorities to benefit the heart and reproductive system; barley juice, vitamin B_1, chiefly responsible for the health of the nerves and as a preventative of beri-beri.

We are told further that these seeds also contain niacin and vitamin C. Niacin is a vitamin mainly known and acclaimed for its ability to prevent pellagra, a disease which is characterized by gastro-intestinal disturbances and skin lesions, while vitamin C is necessary to fortify the body against infections and colds.

It is pointed out in the article that not all varieties of corn contain the same beneficial agents. Kernels of maize, a sugary corn, contain more niacin than do kernels of starchier varieties, according to H. J. Teas of the California Institute of Technology at Pasadena.

S. C. Datta and H. N. De, scientists at Dacca University in India have tested seeds of Bengal gram, mung, pea, cowpea, kalai, rice and wheat. Their research, we are told, has shown that during germination of the seed even more niacin is produced; consequently the juice is more beneficial.

Meanwhile in England, other men of science have been trying to develop better methods of extraction. Research scientists Kon, Baude, Mitchell and Kodiceh of the University of Reading, learned that it was difficult, by normal extraction procedures, to obtain all the niacin contained in seeds because the vitamin was so intricately tied in to all the other properties of the seeds. They found, however, that treating the seeds first with alkali achieved the desired results.

Russian Research on Seeds

Russian scientists have by no means been asleep to the possibility of the value of seeds in the human diet. According to the article, Professors Kondrasheva, Pushkinskaya, Povolotskaya, and Skorobogatova of the A. N. Bakh Institute of Bio-chemistry at the Academy of Science in Moscow, have been engaged in the research of seeds. Among all the seeds they have tested, it was found that sunflower seeds contained the most vitamin B_1, and along with barley and wheat seeds, also contained the most niacin. The highest content of riboflavin was released by soybean seeds. Riboflavin is considered essential to a child's growth and is one of the vitamins so necessary for the health of the skin and eyes.

Experiments With the Husks of Seeds

From what we are told, it appears that the husks of the

seeds may also prove valuable in nutrition. L. B. Vagner of the District Science Research Maternity Institute of Kuibyshev, was engaged in a special study of wheat chaff. Mixing the chaff with hot water, he allowed it to stand for a while until substances within the chaff began to soak out. The chaff was then filtered off. According to the article, premature and underweight infants were given this water-extract by Vagner. He didn't seem quite sure just what it was about the chaff that seemed miraculous, but the infants gained so rapidly that it wasn't long before they outweighed the presumably healthier ones.

Antibiotics Found in Seeds

Scientists L. A. Balabanova and B. N. Tsyurupa have found that seeds such as those of the privet, dog rose, white acacia, common ash, and honey locust contain antibiotic substances similar to penicillin.

The seed of the avocado pear, according to scientists Humberto Valeri and Pievo Gallo, also contains antibiotic substances. At the University of California at Berkeley, Peter A. Ark, professor of plant pathology, has found antibiotics in wheat and barley juice.

Diuretics Found in Seeds

A diuretic is usually prescribed when anyone suffers from an accumulation of fluid in the body and excessive swelling due to various diseases of the kidneys, heart or lungs. We are informed that research scientist V. A. Skovronskii found effective diuretics contained in the seeds of caraway, sweet fennel and anise, which the article states are "particularly safe because they are commonly used as spices and flavorings."

Possible Value of Carrot Seed Extract

A carrot seed extract is particularly fascinating to research scientists Agarwal, Sharma, and Dandiya of the Medical College in Jaipur, India. Testing the extract on animals, they found that it depresses respiration and also relaxes the smooth muscles of the intestines and nonpregnant uterus. The scientists feel that the carrot seed extract may prove valuable in treating mental patients and those with intestinal ailments. It is also their belief that the extract may help relieve some of the tenseness experienced by pregnant women during parturition, and consequently would be of value in obstetrics.

Further Value of Seed Extracts

A further use for seed extracts is as a blood agglutinate. We are informed that up to now only serums have been used for this purpose by doctors. When a blood transfusion is required, a blood sample is taken from the patient and a drop of the donor's serum is added to it. The donor's blood cannot be used if the patient's red blood cells form clumps, or agglutinate; otherwise the patient might die. It is essential, therefore, that the physician duplicate the blood types. We are told that substances similar to serum are contained in certain seeds; consequently they too can be used as the test.

At the University of Marburg/Lahn, Germany, M. Krupe has found remarkably powerful agglutinan in *Sophora japonica* seeds. From 39 varieties of *Phascolus* similar substances have been extracted with water by Lily Trabucco Maron of Chile. The extracts are so strong that even when only one part extract is used with 16,000 parts water they still agglutinate red blood cells. The extracts test all A, B, and O types of human blood.

The article closes by saying:

What new and wonderful medicine may evolve from tiny, ordinary seeds can only be guessed at now; but we know for certain that scientists throughout the world are at last ferreting out one more of Mother Nature's fascinating secrets.

Pumpkin Seeds

In China the pumpkin is the symbol of fruitfulness and health, and is called the Emperor of the Garden. Pumpkin takes its name from the Greek word *pepon* which means "cooked in the sun." It is a plant of the gourd family, native to India, but is now naturalized and cultivated in almost every country throughout the world. It has heart-shaped leaves and large blossoms with yellow petals. The vine often grows to a length of ten to twenty feet, while the fruit, depending upon the species, ranges in size from a few inches to 2 feet in diameter. The seeds are small, white and flat, and lie in rows within the fruit.

Medicinal Use of Pumpkin Seeds

It is the seeds of the pumpkin that are believed to yield valuable medicinal properties, and have been used as a folk remedy for centuries, especially for their purported effectiveness in expelling tapeworm and correcting uriary disorders. Occasionally the flesh of the pumpkin was used as a substitute for the seeds in expelling tapeworm.

In the *Dictionary of Materia Medica* by Merat and De Lens, it is mentioned that Dr. Hoarau had reported that in the Isle of France the seeds of a small variety of pumpkin were used to expel tapeworms without fail. In the year 1820, M. Mongeney, a physician of Cuba, published the results of his experiences with the *flesh* of the pumpkin in treating the same disorder. He related how he had discovered the remedy quite by accident and found it to be repeatedly effective. His method of presentation was to instruct the patient to fast in the morning, after which he was given about 3 ounces of the fresh pumpkin in the form of a paste. This was followed at the end of an hour by about 2 ounces of honey. The 2 ounces of honey was repeated twice at intervals of an hour.

It is believed that attention was first directed to the medical value of the plant in this country when it was mentioned in the *Boston Medical and Surgical Journal,* October 1851. It was listed in the 17th edition of the *Dispensatory of the United States,* 1894, as "one of our most efficient and harmless taeniafuges." (A remedy that expels tapeworms.)

In the current issue of *Potter's New Cyclopaedia of Botanical Drugs and Preparations,* [1] we find the following formula regarding the use of pumpkin seeds in expelling tapeworm:

> The patient fasts for a day, and takes a saline cathartic. Then a mixture—made as follows: 2 oz. of seeds are beaten with as much sugar and milk or water added to make 1 pt.—is given in three doses every two hours, and a few hours after the last dose, a dose of Castor Oil is given. The ordinary infusion —1 oz. to 1 pt.—has also been used in urinary complaints and scalding of urine.

The Value of Pumpkin Seeds in Prostate Disorders [2]

Pumpkin seeds have been used for their vitalizing effect upon the prostate gland. This was a folk remedy of the old days, handed down from father to son. It should be of great interest to every member of the male sex since med-

[1] R. C. Wren, F.L.S. (Sir Isaac Pitman & Sons Ltd., Pitman House, Parker Street, Kingsway, London, W.C.2), 1956.

[2] J. I. Rodale, *The Encyclopedia for Heathful Living,* Rodale Books, Inc., Emmaus, Pennsylvania, 1960.

ical science informs us that some difficulty with the prostate gland affects almost every American man over the age of fifty. Physicians explain that during this period of life the prostate gland may swell and cause great difficulty of urination. Eventually it may become impossible to urinate due to pressure of the gland upon the bladder. The accumulation of urine in the bladder may consequently cause infection. The treatments most often employed by doctors are massage and surgery.

A German doctor recently announced a new theory regarding the age-old use of pumpkin seeds in treating prostate gland disorders. In an article entitled *Androgen-Hormonal Curative Influence of a Neglected Plant,* Dr. W. Devrient of Berlin informs us that the reason the prostate gland becomes enlarged is due to the organ's efforts to make up for the loss of the male hormones which have been steadily declining with the advance of age. This is similar to the menopause experienced by women whose production of the female sex hormones slackens during this period. Dr. Devrient says:

> Its presence (enlarged prostate, that is) can be demonstrated in every fourth American once he has reached the age of 52. It is maintained that the number of impotent males in the United States amounts to some two million. This, too, is related to the hormone production of the prostate, although these processes are centrally regulated. In Berlin, two large specializing urological hospitals had to be founded, because the surgical divisions of the existing hospitals were not sufficient. The causes of this trouble are to be sought in false methods of living. The poisoning of the glands with tobacco plays the most important role among them.

The Gypsies' Secret [3]

Dr. Devrient feels that prevention is the best course to

[3] *Ibid.*

follow with regard to the problem of prostate trouble. He mentions that in certain countries where pumpkin seeds are consumed in abundance throughout life, there is pracly no incidence of prostate disorders.

Only the plain people knew of the open secret of pumpkin seeds, a secret which was handed down from father to son for countless generations without any ado. No matter whether it was the Hungarian gypsy, the mountain-dwelling Bulgarian, the Anatolian Turk, the Ukrainian or the Transylvanian German—they all knew that pumpkin seeds preserve the prostate gland and, thereby, also male potency. In these countries, people eat pumpkin seeds the way they eat sunflower seeds in Russia: as an inexhaustible source of vigor offered by Nature.

Investigations by G. Klein at the Vienna University revealed the noteworthy fact that in Transylvania prostatic hypertrophy is almost unknown. Painstaking researches result in the disclosure that the people there have a special liking for pumpkin seeds. A physician from the Szekler group in the Transylvanian mountains confirmed this connection as an ancient healing method among the people. Dr. Bela Pater, of Klausenburg, later published these associations and his own experiences in the Journal, *Healing and Seasoning Plants.*

My assertion of the androgen-hormonal (the male hormone) influence of pumpkin seeds is based on the positive judgment of old-time doctors, but also no less on my own personal observations throughout the years. This plant has scientifically determined effects on intermediary metabolism and diuresis (urination), but these latter are of secondary importance in relation to its regenerative, invigorative and vitalizing influences. There is involved herein a native plant hormone which affects our own hormone production in part by substitution, in part by direct proliferation.

Anyone who has studied this influence among peasant peoples has been again and again astonished

over the effect of this plant in putting off the advent
of old age. My own personal observations in the
course of the last 8 years, however, have been de-
cisive for me. At my own age of 70 years I am well
able to be satisfied with the condition of my own
prostate, on the basis of daily ingestion of pumpkin
seeds, and with that of my health in general. This
beneficial result can also be found among city patients
who are prudent enough to eat pumpkin seeds every
day and throughout life. But one must continue proving this to the city dweller. The peasants of the
Balkans and of Eastern Europe knew of the healing
effects of these seeds already from their forefathers.

Dr. Devrient mentions that of the number of substances that have been found in pumpkin seeds, no one as
yet knows exactly which it may be that is responsible for
the beneficial effects upon the sex organs.

(Pumpkin seeds have been found to be extremely high
in phosphorus, and appear to have a higher content of
iron than any other seeds. They also contain an abundance of B vitamins, a small amount of calcium and vitamin A, and about 30 percent protein and about 40 percent fat, which is rich in unsaturated fatty acids).

Sesame Seeds

This herb is native to India but is cultivated in many
parts of the world. It grows to a height of from 2 to 3
feet, and bears yellowish or pinkish flowers. The plant
contains seeds which are eaten as food, and which also
yield a pale yellow emollient oil. In India, the oil is used
for anointing as well as for cooking. Turkey exports a
thick cream, made from sesame seeds, which is called
tahini, and is used as a spread or dressing.

Sesame seeds are rich in vitamins, minerals, and protein. They contain an abundance of calcium, and their
content of lecithin makes them a valuable aid in prevent-

ing cholesterol from collecting in the blood. In the various medical systems of India, the seeds are used particularly for the treatment of piles and constipation.

Sunflower Seeds

The botanical name of this plant, *Helianthus annuus,* comes from the Greek words *Helios,* the sun, and *anthos,* a flower. As though magnetized by the sun's rays, the disc of the sunflower follows the great solar orb in its course around the heavens. As the sun rises in the morning, the sunflower slowly faces east. The sunflower not only changes direction but also turns upward, keeping face to face with the sun as it climbs higher in the sky. The flower follows the westward direction of the sun in the afternoon, gradually drooping as the sun begins to set. Evening finds the disc of the sunflower completely facing downward. The entire process is again repeated with the rising of the sun on the following morning.

As Moore so picturesquely stated:

> The sunflower turns on her god when he sets,
> The same look which she did when he rose.

About three centuries ago when Champlain and Segur visited the Indians on the eastern shores of Lake Huron, they saw them cultivating the plant. It is believed that the Indians obtained it from its native prairies beyond the Mississippi. The Redmen highly valued the plant whose stalks provided them with a textile fibre, its leaves fodder, its flowers a yellow dye, and most important of all, its seeds for food and hair oil.

At one time it was thought that the species was native to Peru and Mexico because the Spanish conquerors found it in use there as a sacred and mystic symbol. The Incas worshipped it as a representation of the sun. In the temples, during religious ceremonies, the seeds were eaten and a large sunflower made of pure gold adorned the breasts of the priestess of the sun. The sunflower is the floral emblem of Peru and the State Flower of Kansas.

In Russia, the plant has assumed considerable economic importance. The finest quality of seed is used for food, and is regarded as a delicacy by all classes. The oil is considered highly nutritious and is employed for culinary and domestic purposes. From the cheaper quality of seeds, oil cakes are made and used as a fodder for cattle and horses. The stalks, when burned, produce a brilliant, aromatic fire, and are used as fuel. The ashes also have commercial value for fertilizing purposes. In China, fabrics are made from the fibre of the stalks.

In 1901, under the direction of the Department of Agriculture, Dr. Harvey W. Wiley issued a bulletin on the cultivation, use and composition of the plant. According to the bulletin, the seeds were in demand for keeping cattle and horses in top physical condition. The plant is also mentioned as a preventative of malaria.

Nutritive Value of Sunflower Seeds

Sunflower seeds contain valuable nutritive elements. The oil made from them is excellent as a source of unsaturated fatty acids, ideal for use in salads, cooking, etc. Scientists have found that sunflower seed oil is a valuable aid in reducing the cholesterol level in the blood. The seeds contain a marvelous abundance of vitamins and minerals. They are remarkably rich in the vitamin B complex and are an excellent source of protein. Their high content of phosphorus and calcium makes them a valuable aid in building strong bones and teeth. They also contain carotene, the pro-vitamin A, which science tells us is necessary for the health of the eyes.

Medicinal Value of Sunflower

Because of their oil, sunflower seeds have been used as a medicinal remedy. A medical herbal [4] written by Dr. George P. Wood and Dr. E. H. Ruddock gives the following account of the value of sunflower seeds:

> A decoction of the seeds of the common sunflower gives great relief, in a great majority of the ordinary cases of bronchitis. . . . It will be found a pleasant and reliable remedy. It has been prepared in the following form, and in some cases it acts better than when given alone. Bruise any quantity of the seeds, and add strained honey, enough to cover them. Simmer for one hour, strain, and when cold, add one teaspoonful of the tincture of bloodroot (herb) to each teacupful of the honey. Dose: a teaspoonful, four or five times daily. Its use requires time and patience.

Sunflower *leaves* have long been used by the inhabitants of the *Caucasus* as a treatment of malarial fevers. The value of the herb in this respect was confirmed by Danzel (Revue de Med. Trop., 1929, 21, 158). The *flowers* and *leaves* made into a tincture when combined with balsamic drugs was recommended by Beldau in the treatment of bronchiataesis. A ten percent tincture of the flowers made with 70 percent alcohol was recommended as a febrifuge by Le Clerc (Presse med., 1930, 948).

Watermelon Seeds

As a folk remedy, watermelon seeds were used for certain disorders of the kidneys and urinary passages. They

[4] *Encyclopedia of Health and Home,* Vitalogy Assoc., Chicago, 1921.

were regarded almost equal in value to pumpkin seeds in their ability to expel tapeworm. Recently, scientists at the Institute for the Advancement of Pharmacists, Kiev, found that a substance is present in watermelon seeds that paralyzes tapeworms and roundworms in cats. We are informed that it is the fatty oil and other components of the kernels and hulls which contains this substance.

VIII

the favorite of the pharaohs

He causeth the grass to grow for the cattle, and herb for the service of man:—Psalms 104:14.

LICORICE *(Glycyrrhiza glabra)* is a perennial herb of which there are several varieties. The root penetrates deeply into the ground, and is the part of the herb that contains an abundance of valuable properties. Licorice is indigenous to Greece, Asia Minor, Spain, southern Italy, Syria, Iraq, Caucasian and Transcaspian Russia, and northern China. From time to time, other countries have produced small quantities of the herb but they are considered negligible as a source of supply.

The word licorice is a corruption of the Greek *glykys* (sweet) and *rhiza* (root), meaning sweet root. The root yields a substance known as glycyrrhizin or glycyrrhizic acid which is 50 times as sweet as sugar cane. Practically all other sweets are known to increase thirst, and in this respect licorice stands unique, having just the opposite effect, that of alleviating thirst.

Licorice Known for Ages

The use of licorice dates back to ancient times. Archaeologists have found great quantities of licorice stored among the fabulous jewelry and art treasures in the 3000-year-old tomb of King Tut. The tombs of other Egyptian kings also contained the valuable herb. The practice of placing licorice in the tombs was to enable the departed spirits of the rulers to prepare a sweet drink called *mai sus* in the next world. It is still a favorite beverage among the Egyptians today.

The Brahmans of India, the Hindus, Greeks, Romans, Babylonians and Chinese all knew of the value of licorice. In ancient Greece and Rome licorice was employed as a tonic, and also as a remedy for colds, coughs and sore throat. The ancient Hindus believed it increased sexual vigor when prepared as a beverage with milk and sugar. The Chinese maintained that eating the root would give them strength and endurance, and also prepared a special tea of it for use as medicine.

The Use of Licorice by the Early Herbalists

In 400 B.C., Hippocrates mentioned the use of licorice. Two hundred years later Theophrastus, "Father of Greek Botany," described it as having "the property of quenching thirst, if one holds it in the mouth; wherefore they say the Scythians, with this and mare's milk cheese, can go for eleven or twelve days without drinking." Nineteen hundred years ago Pliny wrote, "The juice of Liquirice reduced to a thicke consistence, if it be put under the tongue, is singular for to cleare the voice. And therewith, both thirst and hunger may be slaked and allaied."

From Turner's Herbal it appears that licorice was cultivated in England in 1562, and Stow specifically states that "the planting and growing of licorish began about the first-year of Queen Elizabeth." (Licorice was cultivated near the old Pontefract Castle, and today some of the licorice candies of England called Pontefract Cakes are stamped with a picture of this castle).

John Josselyn of Boston in the 16th century lists the plant among the "precious herbs" which had been brought over from England to the New World by the early settlers. The Indians bought it from the white settlers and included it in their own pharmacopoeias.

Nicholas Culpepper, one of the greatest and most popular of the early herbalists, wrote an account of the herb which is given in part as follows:

> Liquorice root, boiled in water with some Maidenhair and Figs, makes a good drink for those who have a dry cough or hoarseness, wheezing or shortness of breath . . . It is also a cleansing agent, and at the same time softening and soothing, and therefore balsamic.
>
> The juice, or extract, is made by boiling the fresh roots in water, straining the decoction, and when the impurities have settled, evaporating it over a gentle heat until it will no longer stick to the fingers. It is better to cut the roots into small pieces before boiling them, as the healing agencies in the root will by that means be better extracted. A pound of liquorice root boiled in three pints down to one quart will be found the best for all purposes.
>
> The juice of the liquorice root is most effective, and may be obtained by squeezing the roots between two rollers. When made with due care, it is exceedingly sweet and of a much more agreeable taste than the root itself.

The Use of Licorice in Various Countries Today

Today, huge quantities of licorice are used for a variety of purposes such as foods, medicine, beverages, confections, etc. In 1952, the United States imported 39,718,304 pounds of licorice root and 645,667 pounds of the liquid extract. The root came from Iraq, Turkey, Russia, Syria, Italy, British East Africa, while the extract was imported mostly from Spain, with a very small amount coming from Japan.

A certain portion of the vast amount of licorice entering the United States is used by drug industries. It is employed in the form of an extract and incorporated in various medicaments by reason of its demulcent and expectorant properties. The powdered root is used in the preparations of pills for the purpose of giving them proper consistency or to coat their surfaces to prevent them from cohering. The use of the extract has almost entirely replaced the powder as a remedial agent.

The largest portion of the huge supply of licorice is used by the tobacco industries as a conditioning and flavoring agent; by the confectionary industry for use in the preparation of a wide variety of candies; the residual material after extraction is used as a stabilizer in the production of foam fire-extinguishers, and as a fertilizer for mushrooms.

During the first World War, large amounts of Chinese licorice root were shipped across the Pacific into the United States when transportation through the Mediterranean was prevented. Chinese licorice extract is said to be used in soy sauce. The practicing Chinese herbalists of today still regard licorice as a healing agent either by itself or as an ingredient in various herbal formulas.

In England, as in many other countries, licorice is used in cough syrups and cough drops. The English also use it to flavor beer and ale. Licorice sherbets are popular in Turkey, while in southern Europe, people consume large amounts of licorice water which they believe to be a good blood purifier. In Belgium and France, many workers in the steel industries drink licorice beverages in place of water.

Further Value of Licorice as a Medicinal Agent

For ages, licorice has been considered medicinally valuable due to its demulcent and expectorant properties. It has the reputation of relieving constipation, and at one time it was common practice to give bedridden patients a glass of the juice to relive congested bowels. In Jamaica. licorice is known as lick weed, and is boiled as a tea and given as a laxative both to adults and youngsters.

In the 17th edition of the U. S. Dispensatory, the value of licorice root is fully covered. Here are a few excerpts:

Liquorice root is an excellent demulcent, well adapted to catarrhal affections, and to irritations of the mucous membrane of the bowels and urinary passages. It is best given in the form of a decoction, either alone, or combined with other demulcents. Before being used, it should be deprived of its cortical part, which is somewhat acrid, without possessing the peculiar virtues of the root. The decoction may be prepared by boiling an ounce of the bruised root, for a few minutes, in a pint of water.

Liquorice is a useful demulcent, much employed in cough mixtures, and frequently added to infusions or decoctions in order to cover the taste or obtund the acrimony of the principal medicine. A piece of it held in the mouth and allowed to dissolve slowly is often found to allay cough by sheathing the irritated membrane of the fauces.

In the current edition of *Potter's New Cyclopaedia of Botanical Drugs and Preparations,* [1] licorice is classified as demulcent, pectoral and emollient. It is mentioned as being a popular and well known remedy for chest complaints and coughs. We are told that:

Beach mentions the following recipe as being used by the late Dr. Malone, of London, and speaks most highly of its efficacy—

[1] R. C. Wren, F.L.S. (Sir Isaac Pitman & Sons Ltd., Pitman House, Parker Street, London, W.C.2).

Take a large teaspoonful of Linseed (flaxseed), 1 oz. of Liquorice root, and ¼ lb of best raisins. Put them into 2 qt of soft water and simmer down to 1 qt. Then add to it ¼ lb of brown sugar candy and a tablespoonful of white wine vinegar or lemon juice. Drink ½ pt when going to bed and take a little whenever the cough is troublesome. N.B. It is best to add the vinegar to that quantity which is required for immediate use.

Licorice and Smoking

In *Fads of an Old Physician,* Keith wrote, "Many years ago, when visiting in East Lothian, a Doctor told me he had found Licorice very useful in a way I had not known. Many farm servants who smoked strong tobacco could not look at breakfast until they had a smoke. This was always relieved by taking a bit of Licorice on getting up. . . ."

An interesting experience related by a medical doctor appeared in the 1964 issue of the *Herbalist Almanac:* [2]

Your company was referred to me. I want some licorice root for an unusual purpose. For 25 years I have examined young men for employment in a large baking company, most of whom are cigarette smokers who would like to quit but can't seem to do so. Acting on a hunch that humans like something, nervously, to chew on, a leftover from the time we were babies and had to have something to suck on, I hit upon liquorice root. It has worked so well that I keep it on hand for this purpose.

Scientific Research on Licorice

In recent years, licorice has attained prominence as an agent of potentially great therapeutic value. In Denmark,

[2] Indiana Botanic Gardens, Hammond, Indiana.

experiments have shown it to be effective in the treatment of duodenal and gastric ulcers (Revers. Nederlandsch Tijdscrift v. Geneeskunde, 1948, 92, 2968).

Another valuable property found in licorice root is the female hormone. The following article appeared in the *Science Digest,* June 1950:

> A remedy sold at drug stores and used each month by thousands of women for so-called female trouble now turns out to have real estrogenic (female hormone) action. It owes this, at least in part, to the licorice used to flavor the remedy.
>
> Discovery of the female hormone action of licorice is reported by Christopher H. Costello of Columbus, Ohio, and Dr. E. V. Lynn of the Massachusetts College of Pharmacy, to the *Journal of the American Pharmaceutical Association.*
>
> Three other plant extracts which are ingredients of the remedy also contain estrogenic material. These three are asclepius, helonias, and aletris. But licorice contains significant amounts of it.
>
> These and other plant sources of the female hormone or related chemicals might furnish a cheaper source of the material than ones now used in medicine, Mr. Costello and Dr. Lynn point out. They have worked out a method for practical isolation of the material from licorice.

IX

strange and mystic plants

*Except ye see signs and wonders, ye will not
believe.—St. John 4:48.*

IN MANY PARTS of the world, numerous plants are invested with a mystical symbolism and held as sacred. Such plants were originally chosen for a variety of reasons, but most generally because of a religious association or for their resemblance to some venerated object. One of the most prominent among these is the "Passion Flower." In some mysterious way, this flower appears to bear an astonishing resemblance to some of the objects associated with the crucifixion. A description of the mystical symbolism of this flower, along with its scientific evaluation in medicine will be fully discussed later in this chapter.

In Hindu religion, two trees, the Bael tree *(Aegle marmelos)* and the Crataeva *(Crataeva religiosa)* have trifoliate leaves and are representative of the Trinity. The fruits, leaves, and root-bark of the Bael tree possess medecinal value, and are employed in the medical systems of India.

The lotus is considered sacred in Egypt, Ceylon, India and China. It is depicted as the floating shell of Vishnu, and the seat of Brahma. The Tibetans adorn their temples and altars with it. In China, the Shing-moo or holy mother, is generally depicted holding a blossom of it in her hand, and most temples have some representation of the plant. In ancient Egypt, bouquets and garlands of lotus were offered to the gods. Guests at social gatherings were presented with one of the flowers and a garland was placed on the head in such a way that a single bud or blossom hung down the center of the forehead. A vase filled with lotus blossoms was frequently placed on a stand before the master of the house.

In Central America, there is an orchid which the natives call *"Flor del Espiritu Santo,"* or "Flower of the Holy Ghost." This plant is held sacred because of the remarkable resemblance to a dove which can be seen in the center of the flower. A beautiful description of this plant was given by J. K. Lord, a naturalist of the last century:

> The blossom, white as Parian marble, somewhat resembles the tulip in form; its perfume is not unlike that of the magnolia, but more intense. Neither its beauty nor fragrance begat for it the high reverence in which it is held, but the image of a dove placed at its center. Gathering the freshly opened flower, and pulling apart its alabaster petals, there sits the dove; its slender pinions droop listlessly by its side; the head inclining gently forward, as if bowed in humble submission, brings the delicate beak, just blushed with carmine, in contact with the snowy breast.

This description brings to mind the "snipe orchis," another flower which displays the curious appearance of a bird.

The oak was venerated by the Gauls, and oak leaves and boughs were used in their religious ceremonies. When the mistletoe was observed growing on the oak, it was regarded as a divine gift and considered especially sacred. It was carefully removed by a golden sickle and caught in a white cloth. A beverage was made from the plant and used as an antidote for poisons and a remedy for diseases. It was also believed to insure fertility.

Leaves of Peace

The olive leaf or branch is regarded almost universally as a symbol of peace. There is no way of knowing to what extent this may be due to the Biblical record of the dove returning to the Ark bearing a fresh olive leaf in its beak. It is almost certain that Noah would have regarded it symbolic of the Earth resurrected in peace after the devastation of the flood.

The Great Seal of the United States, which is carried on the one dollar bill, shows the eagle holding an olive branch in its right claw and 13 arrows in the left. This signifies that peace and good will is first and foremost in the heart of our country, and combat only as a last resort for defense.

The "Earthman"

One of the plants that has gathered a mass of legend and tradition is the mandrake. From the earliest periods it was held in veneration in Eastern lands. The root is often forked and in such instances bears a slight resemblance to the shape of a man. (This plant is not to be confused with ginseng whose root also resembles the figure of a man.)

Most of the legends and superstitions associated with mandrake are unpleasant. It was believed that it clung so desperately to the ground that when it was uprooted it groaned and shrieked like a tormented human, causing instant death to anyone hearing it. It is very difficult to imagine that people actually believed such utter nonsense. Evidently it did not occur to them to ask just how it was possible for those hearing the death-dealing cries to convey this warning to others. Legends state that "one must stop his ears carefully, and having tied a dog to the root, run away. The dog is then called, and pulling up the root is instantly killed."

Shakespeare makes several allusions to this superstition about the mandrake. In *Romeo and Juliet,* he writes:

And shrieks like Mandrakes torn out of the earth,
That living mortals hearing them run mad.

And in another instance:

Would curses kill as doth the Mandrake's groan?

The root, or portions of it, were sold as charms, oracles, or as a protection against evil and diseases. Usually the root was secretly carved so that it bore a more perfect resemblance to the shape of a human. The image was given the name of "earthman" and as much as 25 to 30 ducats of gold were paid for one of these artificial charms.

Gerard (1545-1611), an herbalist of early times, endeavored to convince the people that they were being duped and reports that both he and his servant had frequently uprooted a mandrake and heard no death screams. He also adds, "I never saw any such thing upon or in them, as are upon the peddlers' roots that are commonly sold in boxes."

In spite of Gerard's pleas, the majority of people still continued with these superstitious beliefs and as late as 1810 images of the root were still offered for sale in several of the seaport towns in Europe.

Mandrake contains medicinal properties and is generally cited as a strong purgative. Large doses are poisonous.

Plant Emblems of the Virgin Mary

Both the red and white rose, as an emblem of the Virgin Mary, appears at a very early period. This flower was especially recognized by St. Dominic when he instituted the devotion of the rosary with direct reference to the Holy Mother, and it is believed that the prayers were symbolized as roses.

A legend is told of a "lordsman who had gathered much goods of his lords, and who had to pass with his treasure through a wood in which thieves were waiting for him. When he entered the wood, he remembered that he had not that day said 'Our Lady's saulter'; and, as he knelt to do so, the Virgin came and placed a garland on his head and at each ave she set a Rose in the garland that was so bright that all the wood shone thereof. He was himself ignorant of it; but the thieves saw the vision, and allowed him to pass unharmed."

The Rose of Jericho has been called St. Mary's rose, and legends state that when Joseph and the Virgin were fleeing from Herod a rose sprang up to mark every spot where they rested.

Roses occupied a prominent place in the materia medica of the past. Oils, conserves, and other preparations made from the plant, leaves, petals and hips were used in over 32 different remedies, e.g., nervousness, headaches, indigestion, etc. An enchanting perfume called Attar of Roses was also made from the oil.

The white lily, regarded as an emblem of purity and beauty is also devoted to the Madonna. In certain festivals commemorating the journey taken by Mary to visit her cousin Elizabeth, a vase containing three white lilies is placed beside a statue of the Virgin. It is claimed that this practice was adopted in consequence of the miraculous appearance of three lilies to confirm the faith of a master of the Dominican monks.

The marigold is another of the many flowers consecrated to the Virgin. Its name was given because of the resemblance of the florets of its disc to "rays of glory."

Plant Emblems of the Saints

During the Middle Ages, a favorite flower was usually consecrated to, or named after, a saint, especially if the plant was believed to possess medicinal properties. The choice of the saint was usually determined by the month in which the flower bloomed. Most of the names were probably given by the monks who developed gardens and were skilled in the medicinal use of herbs.

St. John's Wort blossoms on St. John's Day, and was believed to possess magical properties. It was gathered and hung in houses as a protection against thunder and evil spirits. The red spots on this herb are said to appear on the 29th of August, the day on which St. John the Baptist was beheaded. Various healing properties are attributed to different species of the plant, generally as astringent, diuretic and expectorant. The flowers are infused in olive oil and applied to wounds, bruises, etc.

The Great Candlestick (*Candelabrum ingens*) was also dedicated to St. John who was a "burning and shining light."

The golden sunflower was introduced as a representation of St. John the Evangelist. In a stained glass window of the Church of St. Remi at Rheims, St. John and the Virgin appear at each side of the cross. Their heads, encircled by aureoles of sunflowers are turned toward the true light of the Christ.

Sunflower seeds contain valuable nutritive elements. According to science, the oil is effective in reducing the cholesterol content in the blood.

In old herbals, the cowslip used to be called St. Peter's Wort due to the fact that the cluster of blossoms somewhat resemble a bunch of keys. Keys were associated with Peter because the Lord addressed him with the words, *"And I will give unto thee the keys of the kingdom of heaven."* Mat. 16:19.

The water fern is connected with St. Christopher who is usually depicted wading through a stream carrying the Infant Christ on his shoulders.

Mystical Plants and the Crucifixion

There is an astonishing number of traditions relating to flowers, plants, or trees associated with the crucifixion. Ancient legends claim that the Libyan Thorn was the plant from which the Savior's crown was made, and is called Christ's Thorn. In France and England this reputation was given to the Whitethorn or Hawthorn. Others claim that it was the Barberry which also bore the name of Holy Thorn. (Herbalists maintain that the Hawthorn is effective as a heart tonic. Recent investigations by science tend to support this belief.)

The cross itself has been said to "fling its shadow over the whole vegetable world" so great is the variety of trees from which it was reputedly made. Some maintain that the aspen supplied the material for the cross and that its leaves have trembled ever since in commemoration of the awesome event.

Others claim that it was the Elder, and this tree has enjoyed a sacred reputation ever since. In early times, a German peasant would pray in front of an Elder tree before wielding the axe. An early writer mentions that once when instructing a number of English children about the dangers of standing under a tree during a thunder storm, he was told by one of them that all trees were not dangerous. "You will be quite safe under an Elder tree," the youngster said, "because the cross was made of that, and so lightning never strikes it."

This same writer says that later he came across a provincial paper which carried the following remarks: "This notion that an elder tree is safe from the effects of lightning, whether true or not, received confirmation a few days ago, when the electric fluid struck a thorn bush in which an Elder had grown up and became intermixed, but which escaped perfectly unscathed, though the thorn was completely destroyed."

The Elder has been used in folk medicine for ages. The Indians made a tea of the flowers as a remedy for colic. Many people believed that the berries were a good blood purifier when eaten as marmalade. Elder tea was used as a diurtic. The berries are employed in making wine and are also prepared as food, especially in the form of pies and jellies.

Other traditions state that the Cedar, Pine, Fir and Box were the four kinds of wood from which the cross was made. This belief was based on the words of Isaiah: *The glory of Lebanon* (i.e., the cedar) *shall come unto thee, the fir tree, the pine tree, and the box together, to beautify the place of my sanctuary.—Isa. 60:13.* The four kinds of wood were symbolic of the four corners of the globe.

Among the gypsies, the cross was believed to be made of oak, while still another belief existed that it was made of cypress. Many other conjectures have been made regarding the particular tree whose wood furnished the material for the cross.

Passion Flower

Many flowers and plants display some resemblance to the crucifixion and are considered highly mystical in various countries. In Rome, there was a gourd called "Zucca" which grew in the garden of a Cistercian convent of Santa Potentiana. When the fruit was cut in half a green cross appeared inlaid on the white pulp. At its angles were five seeds which represented the five wounds.

As mentioned earlier in the chapter, one of the most

prominent of the mystical flowers traditionally associated with the crucifixion is called the Passion Flower *(Passiflora incarnata).* This flower is a handsome climber and regarded as one of the most graceful and lovely plants that can be employed for covering trellises and arbors.

There are several species, some of which produce edible fruits and are used for food or juices in their native countries. Most of the species of Passion Flower are native to the West Indies and the southern part of the United States. In their native habitat they often climb to the tops of the highest trees where they sustain themselves by means of tendrils, and send out an abundance of the most beautiful white and purple flowers. The Spanish friars in America were the first to call it the "flower of passion" as they saw in it a representation of some of the objects associated with the crucifixion. Monardes, a physician and botanist of the 16th century, wrote the first account of the flower and its symbolic interpretation. Shortly afterwards the plant was cultivated in Rome and from there it was believed introduced into Belgium.

Parkinson[1] mentions the plant under the name of *Maracoc sive clematis virginiana,* the Virginia climber, because as he says, "Unto what other family or kindred I might better conjoin it I know not." He considered it "the passing delight of all flowers."

Mystical Symbolism of Passion Flower

The old Spanish missionaries attributed the following symbolism to passion flower:

In the central receptacle, the pillar (column) of the cross may be observed. The corona represents the crown of thorns or halo which surrounded the Lord's head, while the five red spots on each of the leaves are symbolic

---

[1] One of the prominent early herbalists.

of the five wounds. The ten petals are suggestive of the ten apostles, excluding Judas who betrayed Christ and Peter who denied Him. The five anthers are emblematic of the hammers, and the three stigmas represent the three nails which pierced the Saviour's hands and feet. The tendrils are suggestive of the cords or whips, while the small seed vessel is the sponge filled with vinegar which was offered to quench the Lord's thirst. The digitate leaves typify the hands of the persecutors.

When the flower is not entirely opened, it resembles a star and represents the Star of the East seen by the Three Wise Men. The leaves, triplicate in form, testify to the Trinity, and the purple flowers suggest the purple robe that was placed on Him in mockery. The white flowers refer to the purity and light of the Saviour. Because the plant is a vine, it requires support and implies that the aspiring Christian needs the support of the Lord's strength. The loneliness of Christ is typified by the flowers which grow singly on each stem.

Medicinal Use of the Passion Flower

Passion flower was an ancient herbal sedative, antispasmodic and nervine, and is still used as such in various parts of the world today. It is considered a reliable remedy in treating nervous disorders, insomnia, hysteria, etc. In Paris, in 1927, it was shown by Dr. Leclerc that the herb had a calming effect on nervous restlessness, particularly during convalescence and the menopause. Many years of use and experiments have shown that it neither results in disorientation nor depression.

Swinburne Clymer, M.D., mentions the following in his book *Nature's Healing Agents:* [2]

Passion Flower: It is an antispasmodic and mild

[2] Quakertown, Pa.: The Humanitarian Society, Reg., 1960.

soporific. It is indicated in asthenic insomnia, and in some cases of infantile spasms and also in the restlessness and insomnia of low fevers. It is given by Physio-Medicalists in cases usually placed under bromides.

Passiflora should be given in all feverish conditions where there is extreme nervousness and lack of sleep. It is quieting and soothing to the nervous system. The Nature physician refuses to give drugs that are habit forming. *Passiflora* takes the place of narcotics.

Dr. Clymer also quotes information given by another doctor on the medicinal use of passion flower:

. . . It is useful in controlling asthenic insomnia, particularly of childhood and old people. When in typhoid and other adynamic fevers the patient is extremely restless and excitable and cannot sleep, this agent will give rest and slowly produce a remarkably natural and refreshing sleep. It is especially valuable for asthenic conditions; when these are present it tones the sympathetic nervous system, improving the circulation and nutrition of the nerve centers. —Dr. Neiderkorn—*Lloyd's*.

Dr. Clymer recommends that, "Passiflora should be combined with other agents indicated in nervousness and nervous irritation due to many and various causes. Dose of the Tincture (should be made only of the green herb) 5 to 60 drops."

In speaking of combining Passion Flower with *other agents*, Dr. Clymer is referring to other herbs that are also reputed to have sedative properties. For example he mentions the following:

In insomnia or exhaustion whether from excessive application to business or due to alcoholics combine:
Tinc. Scutellaria (Scullcap) 1 oz.
Tinc. Passiflora (Passion Flower) 1 oz.

Dose 20 to 60 drops in water as required.

In another instance he remarks about the virtues of Lady's Slipper herb as a nerve medicine, and states, "It does well combined with Passiflora when there is great restlessness and irritability."

An English Doctor's Report on Passion Flower

An interesting article written by Dr. Eric Powell appeared in an English publication, *Fitness and Health From Herbs*, March 1964. It is quoted in part as follows:

> This precious plant has been described as the remedy that brings peace to mind and body. Acting through the brain and nervous system it relaxes where there is muscular or organic tension, eases pain (pain is always associated with tension and contraction) and promotes a state of calmness throughout the entire organism. We have found it is of great value in spasmodic conditions, nervous headaches, neuralgia, hysteria and high blood pressure when due to mental nervous causes. What is not generally known is that Passion Flower is an eye tonic and a very good one. In some cases it surpasses Eyebright as a remedy for inflamed eyes and dimness of vision. According to Dr. Guyon Richards it kills a form of bacteria that causes eye irritation.

Entire Herbal Nervine Scientifically Developed [3]

It has recently been announced that a new daytime herbal sedative called *Biral,* made by Dr. Madaus & Co., has been introduced into England. The formula was developed in Germany and contains the active ingredients of five herbal plants, one of which is Passion Flower. The plants are given in their official terms and are listed as

[3] Fitness And Health From Herbs, March 1964.

Corydalis cavo, Centranthus ruber, Valeriano officinalis. Avena sativa and *Passiflora incarnata*. Many years of experiment and clinical research on the sedative properties of numerous plants has resulted with the formulation of this product.

It is reported that the product lessens the sensitivity of the central nervous system without in any way "impairing the powers of concentration," which are so much in evidence with the use of most sedatives, such as depression, fuzziness, tiredness and other side effects. This makes it value exceptional as a daytime sedative for mental tension associated with the daily stress and pressures of "modern living."

The report further states that "It has an inhibitory action on the hypersensibility of both constitutional and mental origin. This is especially so when the autonomic nervous system is stressed, as shown in the frequent changes of the color of the skin, anxiety feelings and tendency to sweating." We are also informed that the herbal is particularly effective in cases of occupational strain and severe mental stress, including that of stage fright and the apprehension of examinations.

Properties Contained in the Herbal Sedative

As we have already considered the virtues of Passion Flower, we may briefly examine the remaining four plants included in the new daytime herbal formula.

For many generations in the Mediterranean countries, *Centranthus ruber* has been used as a sedative in folk medicine. That it has never been known to produce any side effects was pointed out by Sabatini as far back as 1939.

Valeriana officinalis is perhaps one of the best known herbal sedatives. Gstirner and Kind, in 1951, showed that the effect of the herb's properties was caused by the cooperation of several active principles.

Another well known mild sedative is *Avena sativa,* and its efficacy was demonstrated by Kroeber, Bohn and Schulz in Germany in 1947, 1935, and 1929 respectively. The plant contains magnesium, manganese and calcium. It also contains a high content of organic phosphorus.

The bulb of *Corydalis cavo* contains *bulbocapnin* and has long been used for its effectiveness in treating nervous irritability. In 1936, Pichler showed that this combined very well with other sedatives to promote agreeable conditions of relaxation.

In America

In our own country, some of the sleeping pills and nerve sedatives which are sold in drug stores without a prescription contain Passion Flower as one of their main ingredients. These drugs are advertised as non-habit forming. Of the tablets containing the herb, you will find Passion Flower listed among the ingredients as *Passiflora incarnata* which is the botanical name of the plant.

X

the medicine tree

For the tree of the field is man's life.
—Deu. 20:19.

THE PAPAYA IS a tropical melon-like fruit which is produced in clusters by the *Carica papaya* tree. The tree, which grows to a height of 20 feet, is crowned by a tuft of leaves on long footstalks and is related to the passion flower family. Papaya is not too well known on the mainland of the United States, but is extensively used in Hawaii and is of major importance in Asia and Africa.

In the tropics, fascinating stories and legends are told of the papaya tree where it has been valued as a food and medicine for ages. In certain regions it is regarded by the natives as a mystical plant because in some ways it appears to possess human attributes, producing male and female flowers on separate plants, while the fruit, like the human embryo, develops in about nine months.

Although it is mainly tropical in its requirements, repeated efforts have been made to extend the tree to subtropical areas. On the mainland of the United States it is produced in limited quantities almost entirely in southern Florida. Recently, however, attempts have been made to grow the plant on a commercial basis in the lower Rio Grande Valley of Texas.

Common Names of Papaya

Papaya is often referred to as The Medicine Tree or Melon Tree. In the West Indies, it is called Pawpaw or papaw, and this name has been adopted by many English-speaking countries as a synonym for papaya. This is apt to cause some confusion, however, as there is a small shrub or tree *(Asimina triloba)* of North America which also bears the name Pawpaw. The latter is a member of the custard-apple family and is not related to papaya.

Papaya Known to the Early Explorers

Papaya is frequently mentioned in the writings of the early explorers. Columbus was deeply impressed by the fact that the natives of the Caribbean could eat exceptionally heavy meals of fish and meat without any apparent distress if the meal was followed by a dessert of papaya. Marco Polo credited the fruit with saving the lives of his sailors when they were stricken with scurvy. According to Ponce de Leon, natives called it Vanti, a word that meant "keep well," and Vasco da Gama referred to papaya as the Golden Tree of Life. Magellan regarded it as a valuable article of the diet.

Many of the ancient explorers also observed that the natives could tenderize tough meat or fowl by wrapping it in green papaya leaves overnight before cooking. Sometimes the juice or slices of the unripe fruit were simply rubbed over the meat, which served the same purpose. In the tropics these practices are still employed today.

Papaya as a Health Food

The golden ripe papaya melon has a pleasant and unique taste and is generally recognized as a valuable health food. It is an excellent source of vitamin A, a good source of vitamin C, and also contains vitamins B and G. It is used in a variety of ways, sometimes served alone and eaten in the same manner as the cantaloupe, or made into sherbets, fruit cocktails, salads, marmalades or jam. The preserves generally include the addition of other flavoring agents such as lemon juice or ginger. The green fruit is often stewed or baked, and used as a substitute for squash. Papaya is also put up in the form of a bottled drink.

Because the fruit is highly perishable, importations from tropical regions into the United States has been a problem. Recently, however, arrangements have been made to ship the melons from Hawaii by jet planes, and the papaya may become a popular health fruit among the people on the mainland.

Further Value of the Papaya

Almost every part of the papaya tree is believed to contain medicinal properties. The unripe fruit as well as other parts of the plant contain a powerful protein-digesting enzyme called papain which greatly resembles pepsin in its digestive action. The crude papain of commerce is obtained by slashing the green fruits while they are still on the tree. The collected latex is allowed to evaporate in porcelain-lined containers until a granular residue results, which is then purified and dried at a low temperature.

The natural papain enzyme extracted from the unripe papaya melon has found employment in medicine, industry, and as a meat tenderizer. It is also made into tablets and sold as a valuable aid for protein digestion. Doctors inform us that as we grow older, the secretion of the natural juices in our bodies often declines, causing incomplete digestion. This can result in gas, bloating, heartburn and stomach discomfort. These unpleasant symptoms may also occur among younger people whose digestion is disturbed by a sense of hurry, frustration, stress, etc. Papaya enzyme tablets aid in digesting the proteins of eggs, milk, meat, beans and similar food products.

Papain is also valued as an active blood clotting agent and has been employed to arrest bleeding. It is also said to be effective in destroying intestinal worms.

Digestive Enzymes Found in Other Botanicals

Many plants and fruits besides papaya also contain protein-digesting enzymes; however, few are known in which the quantity of the enzyme is as great. Recently a meat-digesting enzyme called bromelin was found in appreciable quantities in the juice of the pineapple. This substance is similar to papain and though there are slight differences in action it appears that it would serve the same purpose.

Whereas the *unripe* papaya contains the largest quantity of latex, while the *ripe* yields only minute amounts and is almost devoid of the papain enzyme, ripening does not destroy the bromelin in the pineapple. This explains why pineapple juice cannot be made into gelatin desserts, since gelatin is protein and is digested by the enzyme contained in pineapple juice. This may also account for the fact that the popular home remedy of using fresh pineapple or the juice for relieving a sore throat has been steadfastly maintained for so many years. The dead tissues would be digested by the enzyme, but the live healthy tissues would be comparatively unaffected.

Variety of Uses of Papain [1]

Importations of papain coming from British East Africa, Belgian Congo, Ceylon and Thailand amounted to 282,432 pounds during the year 1952.

[1] *The Dispensatory of the United States of America,* 25th Ed.

A considerable amount of papain imported into the United States is used for tenderizing meat. The enzyme may be rubbed on or mixed with the meat just before cooking. The tanning industry uses papain for batting hides and skins. The latex is employed in the manufacture of chewing gum. As previously mentioned, papaya enzyme tablets are marketed for their excellent ability to aid in the digestion of proteins.

It is estimated that about 80 percent of American beer is treated with papain for making the beverage "chill proof." The enzyme digests the proteins which would otherwise precipitate on cooling, and consequently cause the beer to become cloudy.

For the prevention of post-operative adhesions, scientists prepared a sterile solution of papain which was employed with good results in a large number of patients.[2] Physicians have also applied it topically in the following disorders: Sloughing wounds,[3] carbuncles,[4] burns,[5] dissolving the membrane of diphtheria,[6] and for clearing the discharge of the middle ear.[7]

Remedial Use of the Papaya Tree in Other Countries

The following excerpts on the use of the papaya tree are taken from the book *Medicinal Plants of India and Pakistan:*

The leaves are anthelmintic and febrifuge; they

[2] *Dispensatory of the United States of America*, 25th Ed., pg. 1783, 1st para.: Ochsner and Storck, *Ann. Surg.*, 1936, 104, 736; Donaldson, *Arch. Surg.*, 1938, 36, 20; Elliott and Meleny, *Surgery*, 1937, 1, 785.

[3] *Ibid.*: Glasser, *Am. J. Surg.*, 1940, 50, 320.

[4] *Ibid.*: Garcin, *Gaz. Med. de France*, 1936, 43, 1021.

[5] *Ibid.*: Cooper *et al.*, *Am. J. Dis. Child.*, 1943, 65, 909.

[6] *Ibid.*: deGoldfiem, *Presse med.*, 1934, 42, 387.

[7] *Ibid.*: Tremble, *Can. Med. Assoc. J.*, 1939, 40, 149.

are given in beri-beri; they contain the alkaloid carpaine which physiologically has the same effect as digitalis; . . . Lightly bruised roasted leaves are applied as a galactogogue to breasts of nursing mothers; an application of hot leaves relieves pains . . .

The ripe fruit is alterative, cholagogue, stomachic, appetizer, digestive and antiscorbutic; it is given in piles and enlarged liver and spleen; the ripe fruit is eaten regularly for habitual constipation and chronic diarrhea.

The juice being an irritant is applied to swellings to prevent suppuration, . . . and to corns, warts, pimples, horny excrescences of the skin and other skin diseases; the juice, as a cosmetic, removes freckles and makes the skin smooth and delicate.

The seeds contain the glucoside caricin; they are anthelmintic, emmenagogue and carminative; for expelling roundworms they are given with honey; their juice is given in dyspepsia, bleeding piles, and enlargement of the liver and spleen . . . A paste of the seeds is applied to skin diseases like ringworm.

XI

citrus fruits

My fruit is better than gold, yea, than fine gold;
—Pro. 8:19.

SCIENTIFIC RESEARCH has established the fact that citrus
fruits are very important food factors in the well-balanced
diet. Records show that some of the ancients had an ink-
ling of this truth, and believed that these fruits possessed
valuable health and medicinal properties. A monograph,
thought to be one of the earliest scientific treatises on the
citrus fruits, was presented by Han Yen-chih, a Chinese
writer of the 12th century. In it he stated that the peel of
the Chu (orange) was very good when prepared and used
as a tonic.

Ferrarius, a Jesuit who lived in Rome in 1646, was
also among the first to write about the citrus fruits. He
recorded some interesting beliefs about the orange which
were current in his day. A fermentation of orange flowers
was used as a remedy for the heart, while a water prepared from the orange itself was remedial for "pestilent
fevers accompanied by eruptions." Sneezing could be pro-
voked by a snuff made from the rind and was used to
clear the head. Orange marmalade, similar to that of

126

modern times, was given to older people as an appetizer. Distilled water prepared from the flowers was said to be of "joyous odor and good for a sluggish stomach."

The Lemon

The lemon tree was originally a native of the tropical regions of India and Burma, where they have grown wild since prehistoric times. Between A.D. 900 and 1000, they spread from Persia to Egypt and Palestine and were introduced into Spain by the Arabs around the 12th century. It is believed that the returning Crusaders brought lemons as well as limes and oranges to Europe, and records show that by the middle of the 13th century these fruits were well known in Italy.

Lemons were introduced into the Western hemisphere when Columbus stopped at one of the Canary Islands in October of 1493, gathering seeds of the citrus fruits as well as other plants which he brought with him on his second trip to the New World. Early in the 16th century, the Spanish conquerors carried the seeds of these fruits to the mainland of Mexico and Central America. They were planted in St. Augustine, Florida, in 1565 when the Spanish settled there. Two centuries later, the seeds were brought to California by the Franciscan Fathers when they moved from Mexico.

The lemon tree has since been naturalized and many highly improved species have been produced by cultivation. They are grown in large orchards in the warmer regions of America and Europe, especially in the islands and countries of the Mediterranean. The cultivation of the lemon was introduced into Australia in 1790.

Favorite Species of Lemons

Among the favorite species of lemons are the citron lemon, thick-skinned lemon, sweet lemon and common lemon. They are principally used for flavoring in cookery, lemonade and other drinks, medicine, and the manufacture of oil of lemon. Oil of lemon is obtained from the rind by pressure and is so potent that a few drops will flavor 50 gallons of water.

Lemons as Medicine

Of all foods which have also been used as medicines, lemons are the most commonly known. The custom of using a slice of lemon when eating a fish dinner was originally intended for remedial purposes rather than for flavoring. It was believed that if a fish bone were to be unknowingly swallowed during the meal, the juice of the lemon would dissolve it.

As a domestic remedy, lemons have been employed in a variety of ailments such as colds, rheumatism, sore throat, headache, heartburn, biliousness, etc. Drinking lemonade at intervals is a favorite in many lands for the relief of hiccoughs. The application of lemon juice mixed with glycerine is used for chapped lips or chilblains. For constipation, the juice of a lemon is taken in a glass of hot water one-half hour before breakfast. Local applications of lemon juice are used to allay the irritation caused by the bite of gnats and similar insects.

Lemon Powder

During the second World War, submarine crews of the British navy were given citrus concentrates as a supplement to their diets. German soldiers were supplied with a lemon-pectin powder and told to sprinkle it over their wounds, as it was an effective clotting agent. Lemons were used in many of the war-stricken countries to enrich the diets of the undernourished. Russian troops at the front were fed lemon powder. The powder was also distributed to prison camps in Italy, Japan and Germany by the International Red Cross. When climbing Mt. Everest, Sir Edmund Hillary and Tensing Norkay prepared lemonade from lemon powder for use as an energy builder.

Lemons and Scurvy

Lemons were highly valued in former times as a treatment and prevention of scurvy. Scurvy is a disease characterized by a spongy condition of the gums, loosening of the teeth, foul breath, debility and anemia. There is also a tendency to hemorrhage, especially into the mucous membranes and skin.

For ages, Europe was plagued with this dread disease in areas where fresh fruits, greens, or vegetables were either totally excluded from the diet or consumed in such small quantities that their nutritional value was practically worthless. Scurvy was common among the crewmen on the old-time sailing vessels where the diet consisted entirely of dried or salted foods.

When Vasco da Gama made his voyage around the Cape of Good Hope, he lost 160 men from the ravages of scurvy. In 1535, Jacques Cartier, the French explorer and navigator, found himself stranded in the Canadian wilderness when scurvy claimed the lives of one-quarter of his men and left those remaining in such weakened condition that the return voyage was impossible. Compassionate Indians saved the lives of Cartier and his survivors with a concoction made from the needles and twigs of an evergreen tree.

In the year 1700, every ship leaving port for foreign lands was required by English law to carry a supply of lemon or lime juice as a prevention against scurvy. Each seaman was given a daily allowance of an ounce after having been at sea for ten days. It was this use of limes that gave the English sailor the nickname of "limey."

The Scientific Answer to Scurvy

Though it was over two hundred years ago that lemons were recognized as valuable in the prevention of scurvy, it was only recently that science identified the element so necessary to the health of the body. The answer to scurvy was vitamin C, a substance isolated from lemons after a lengthy study of biological oxidation by Dr. Szent-Gyorgi of Hungary. At about the same time as Dr. Szent-Gyorgi published his findings, Dr. Charles King of Pittsburgh, working independently, also announced that he had isolated vitamin C. Similar announcements from other scientists soon followed. (Note: vitamin C is present in many fresh plant foods though some contain a higher amount than others. Citrus fruits are rich sources of vitamin C.)

Value of Bioflavonoids

Through further experimentation, Dr. Szent-Gyorgi discovered that the pure extracted vitamin C, also known as ascorbic acid, did not seem to possess the same healing power as it did in its natural state. As he continued his investigations he learned that other properties, now called bioflavonoids, were mingled with the vitamin C in lemons. These properties, contained especially within the peel, greatly assisted the utilization of vitamin C in the body, and the combination was found effective not only against the skin hemorrhages of scurvy and similar ailments, but seemed valuable in conditions of excessive bleeding in general.

Further experiments by other scientists proved that whatever vitamin C could do alone, it did much better when combined with the bioflavonoids.

Lemons and Radiation

X-ray treatments are employed to arrest cancerous growths in patients; however, its use may adversely affect the living tissues. A few years ago, experiments on rats given cancer transplants were performed at Florida Southern College, Lakeland. The rats were given lemon-peel medicine and then treated with X-ray radiation. The cancers stopped growing, while the healthy tissues remained undamaged. Experiments were then tried on humans at the Harlem Hospital in New York. Doctors gave the lemon compound to several cancerous patients and found that they could withstand much heavier radiation without any damage to healthy tissues, while the tumors were successfully retarded. Other physicians who employed this method also reported the same favorable results. Good reports from several other hospitals were cited in medical journals.

Some scientists feel that the substances in lemons hold promise as a protective agent against the adverse effects of the radioactive fallout of the atom bomb, which causes intestinal bleeding, destruction of the blood corpuscles, etc.

Nutritional Value of the Citrus Fruits

Citrus fruits are rich in vitamin C, and also furnish numerous other vitamin factors, especially vitamin A, inositol, and certain of the B complex. They also supply appreciable supplementary amounts of minerals with which to increase the totals obtained from other foods. Minerals build rich blood, strong bones, nerve tissue, and assist in regulating the body. Calcium found in oranges makes them a valuable food for infants as it is necessary for growing bodies. This is one of the reasons why many physicians also suggest that the diet of nursing mothers include liberal amounts of this fruit.

Bulk is provided by the cellulose of lemons and oranges, and gives them a laxative effect. With the orange, this effect is said to be increased if the white of the peel is also eaten. This is a favorite practice in some of the Mediterranean countries where citrus fruits are grown. The thin outer rind is removed with a sharp knife leaving the white peel intact on the orange so that the fruit and peel may be eaten together.

The readily available carbohydrate of the citrus fruits makes them important in combatting hypoglycemia (low blood sugar).[1] Many doctors recommend an in-between meal "Citrus Snack" as a "pick-up" for growing children, teen-agers, geriatric patients, active adults, and convalescents. In a series of controlled tests, Mack[2] reports that drinking orange juice between meals is significant as a fatigue resistant in children and adults.

Though acid to the taste, citrus fruits have an alkaline reaction in the body and are valuable in balancing the acids of other foods such as eggs, fish, fowl, meats, breads, cereals, etc. A grapefruit eaten at breakfast and a glass of lemonade taken with the other meals is said to aid digestion.

Scientific knowledge concerning the nutritional value of the citrus fruits is continually increasing. In a publication on this subject, Hilbert[3] states: "Whereas 15 years ago we had but a meager idea of the many constituents of oranges, current research is bringing many of the details to light. We now recognize 11 amino acids, 17 carotenoid pigments, of which 4 have vitamin A activity, and 11 flavonoids of which 8 have not as yet been identified. The

[1] Jolliffe, N., and Alpert, E.: *Postgrad. Med.* 9:106, 1951.

[2] Mack, P. B., *et al.*: *Am. Pract. & Digest. Treat.* 6:584, 1955.

[3] Hilbert, G. E.: *Proc. Nat. Food & Nutr. Inst., U.S. Dept. Agri. Handbook No. 56.* 1952, p. 86.

flavoring constituents of the oil are no less than 28 in number. Of course there are many others yet to be found."

Vitamin C

Medical men inform us that an adequate amount of vitamin C in the diet helps to form and maintain collagen. They explain that collagen is a gelatin-like gristle that holds the billions of cells together in the body. It is concentrated in ligaments, joint ends of bones, gum tissues, and the walls of all the blood vessels. It also gives elasticity and strength to the connective tissues. Therefore we are advised that vitamin C is necessary to the normal healing rate of wounds and to prevent bruises from discoloring the skin for too long a period of time. Its function is also to strengthen the body's resistance to infection and maintain tissue integrity of the teeth, bones and gums.

Vitamin C Must be Supplied Daily

Most animals manufacture vitamin C in their own bodies; however, three species, man, monkey and the guinea pig, must get their vitamin C in their food. This is why scientists doing research on the deficiencies of this vitamin experiment with the ape and the guinea pig.

If the body is not supplied with an adequate amount of vitamin C every day and shortages are continued over long periods of time, the gums may become tender and bleed easily, joints may hurt and swell, black and blue marks may appear readily at the very slightest bruise, the chance of hemorrhage which may result from a "stroke" is far greater, and colds may be taken frequently and are often unduly prolonged. Extreme shortages of vitamin C result in the disease known as scurvy.

Daily Requirements of Vitamin C

Although authorities differ as to the normal daily requirements of vitamin C, the recommended dietary allowance agreed upon by the National Research Council is given as follows:

Men	75 mg. daily	
Women	70 " "	
Pregnant Women	100 " "	
Lactating Women	150 " "	
Infants		
1 month to 1 year	30 " "	
Children		
1 to 3 years	35 " "	
4 to 6 years	50 " "	
7 to 9 years.	60 " "	
Boys		
10 to 12 years	75 " "	
13 to 15 years	90 " "	
16 to 20 years	100 " "	
Girls		
10 to 12 years	75 mg. daily	
13 to 15 years	80 " "	
16 to 20 years	80 " "	

VITAMIN C CONTENT IN THE FOLLOWING FRUITS

1 whole orange	75 mg.
4 oz. orange juice	40 to 50 mg.
½ large grapefruit	75 mg.
1 med. tangerine	25 mg.
Lime or lemon juice, 1 Tbsp.	7 mg.

When the Intake of Vitamin C Should Be Increased

Smoking and Alcoholic Beverages. Reports have shown that the greatest damage to the vitamin C content in the humans is from smoking or from drinking of alcoholic beverages. One cigarette destroys 25 mg. of vitamin C in the body, which means that 500 mg. are neutralized for every package of cigarettes smoked. (W. J. McCormick, Arch. of Ped. N.Y. 69:151–166 April 1952).[4]

Assuming that a person does include citrus juices or other plant foods as part of the breakfast, a cigarette smoked directly after will greatly deplete the amount of vitamin C taken with the meal, and the body must endeavor to function normally on a short supply of this essential vitamin.

If smoking is continued throughout the morning, the store of vitamin C will be entirely neutralized. To replace this loss, foods containing ascorbic acid must be consumed during lunch, although this replacement will also be depleted if one continues to smoke for the rest of the afternoon. And, again, even though fruits, juices, or vegetables are added to the dinner meal the vitamin C content which they supply will be destroyed if smoking is continued for the balance of the evening.

So it is obvious that a smoker will always require much more vitamin C than the non-smoker. This may explain why those who smoke generally are more prone to infections than those who do not. According to reports from Mayo Clinic, post-operative pneumonia is four times as great among habitual smokers as non-smokers.

Stress. Stress disorders often impose increased demands for vitamin C. Of the various conditions treated by the

[4] Fred R. Klenner, M.D. & Fred Bartz, *The Key To Good Health—Vitamin C* (Chicago: Graphic Arts Foundation, 1961).

medical profession, it is estimated that at least one-fifth are caused in part by stress.[5] According to a recent publication, some 50 common disorders are attributed to stress, including certain cardiac symptoms, several types of skin diseases, anxiety states, numerous disorders of the alimentary tract, vasomotor disturbances, etc.[6] The discovery of very low blood levels of vitamin C in stress conditions has resulted in the recommendation by many scientists for an increased intake of this vitamin.[7]

Disease, Injuries. Up to ten times the normal requirement of vitamin C for a period of one year or longer is needed in cases of disease or injury.[8] Patients suffering from burns have a greater need for vitamin C which is necessary for tissue regeneration. Prolonged treatment with cortisone or ACTH depletes ascorbic acid from the body[9] and consequently patients using these treatments need increased amounts of this vitamin. The use of antibiotics or barbiturates also induces deficiency of vitamin C.

[5] Gillison, Keith: *Practitioner* 172:190, 1954.

[6] Finlay, B., *et al.: Practitioner* 172:183, 1954.

[7] Bessey, O. A., *et al.: Ann. Rev. Biochem.* 22:573, 1953; Booker, W. M., *et al.: J. Clin. Endocrinol.* 12:346, 1952; Kark, R. M.: in: *Current Therapy* 1954, edited by Howard F. Conn, Philadelphia, W. B. Saunders, 1954, p. 404; Pirani, C. L.: *J. A. M. A.* 153:1467, 1953; Schilling, J. A., *et al.: Surg. Gynec. & Obst.* 97:434, 1953.

[8] Gale, E. T., and Thewlis, M. W.: *Geriatrics* 8:80, 1953; Jolliffe, N.: J. A. M. A. 129:613, 1945; Jolliffe, N.: in: *Clinical Nutrition,* edited by Norman Jolliffe *et al.,* New York, Paul B. Hoeber, 1950, pp. 627-634 and in the same issue, by F. F. Tisdall, and N. Joliffe, pp. 586-601.

[9] Ershoff, B. H.: in: *Vitamins and Hormones,* Vol. 10, edited by R. S. Harris *et al.,* New York, Academic Press, 1952, pp. 107 ff, 128; Holley, H. L., and McLester, J. S.: *Arch. Int. Med.* 88:760, 1951; Stefanini, M., and Rosenthal, M. C.: *Proc. Soc. Exper. Biol. & Med.* 75:806, 1950.

Old Age. Elderly people generally require more vitamin C than younger adults. [10] Cass *et al*.[11] found that the average blood level of ascorbic acid was 0.35 per 100 ml. in studying a group of 40 elderly patients in a hospital which specializes in chronic diseases. This level was increased to well within the normal in one month by adding 8 ounces of orange juice to the daily diet. It was observed that pain decreased somewhat in arthritic patients, and in many cases of multiple scleroses there was a degree of subjective and objective improvment.

Parker and Hines [12] found that large quantities of vitamin C strengthens the capillaries in certain vascular diseases, particularly those with concurrent diabetes.

This point of view is also emphasized by Winfield when he says: "Citrus fruits as a source of vitamin C and other nutrients are a particularly important food for persons whose normal digestive functionings have been disturbed by illness or age. The high vitamin C content of these fruits will not only tend to restore the proper level of the vitamin in the body, but it will militate against further infection and operate to restore tissue and capillary lesions."

The following report on the effects of vitamin C deficiency among the aged appeared in the publication *The Key to Good Health—Vitamin C:* [13]

ALL SENILE PATIENTS LACK VITAMIN C

A senile patient is forgetful, confused, his speech

[10] Winfield, I. W.: *Nursing Home Administrator* 6:5, 1952 and 8:6, 1954.

[11] Cass, L. G., *et al.: Geriatrics* 9:375, 1954.

[12] Hines, L. E., and Parker, R. J.: *Quart. Bull. Northwestern Univ. School* 23:424, 1949.

[13] Fred R. Klenner, M.D. and Fred Bartz (Graphic Arts Research Foundation, Chicago, Ill. 1961).

rambles. He repeats a question that has just been answered. Memory is so poor the individual does not recognize members of his own family.

Dr. Berkenau made a study of "senile dementia" patients at the Warneford Hospital, Oxford, England, in 1940. He found all his patients were short of vitamin C. No exceptions. "A deficit of 1500 milligrams may be regarded as pathological (disease causing)." The "deficit of these patients varied from 2400 to 3000 milligrams."

"Plaques appeared in the brain of senile patients identical to those found in alcoholics. This indicates a poisonous origin. Hence senile patients and those approaching old age need substantial quantities of vitamin C to protect their brain from damage and to fight infections." (P. Berkenau, *J. of Med. Science,* vol. 86, pg. 675, 1940)

Advantages of Natural Vitamin C Over Synthetic Ascorbic Acid

Ascorbic acid alone naturally deserves a place in the prevention and treatment of vitamin C deficiency, however, Chick [14] states that "the juices of citrus fruits may prove to be more efficient and more complete in their action." Jungleblut [15] observed superior clinical results when citrus fruits were used than from vitamin C alone. Other scientists reported that higher levels of vitamin C storage were found in the tissues when the intake was from food sources. [16]

In the citrus fruits, ascorbic acid is always accompanied by a bonus of other necessary nutrients which Nature in her wisdom has supplied. Ascorbic acid, or vita-

[14] Chick, H.: *Nutrition* 7:59 (No. 2) Summer, 1953.

[15] Jungeblut, C. W.: *J. Exper. Med.* 70:315, 1939, through Bauer, von H.: *Helvet, med. acta* 19:470, 1952.

[16] Cotereau, H. *et al.*: *Nature* 161:557, 1948; Hawley, E. E., *et al.*: *J. Nutrition* 14:1, 1937.

min C, is utilized much better when taken in its natural form. For example, in 29 cases of mild scurvy, 300 milligrams of vitamin C were given orally and 26 of the patients responded favorably within 10 days. Three, however, showed no improvement, so injections of vitamin C were used. Still there was no favorable response. Then the juice of 10 lemons was given daily and the symptoms of scurvy disappeared.

Various Citrus Products as a Source of Vitamin C

As a dependable source of vitamin C, the citrus fruits or juices may be used fresh, canned or as fresh-frozen concentrates. Under the customary condition of storage, fresh-frozen concentrates retain their high vitamin C content almost indefinitely.[17] There was no loss of the vitamin after 12 months at a temperature of 10° F. Even at a temperature as high as 40° F for one year, there was 95% retention. When the frozen concentrate is mixed with water more than 94% of its original content of vitamin C is still retained after two days in a household refrigerator at 50° F.[18]

The Council on Foods and Nutrition of the American Medical Association describes fresh-frozen concentrated orange juice as the "nutritive equal" of fresh orange juice, assuming strict adherence to packing and handling procedures.

The vitamin C content is largely retained in the canning of citrus fruits and juices. Procedures that avoid delay in distribution minimize any gradual loss due to storage.

Canned orange and grapefruit juices were found to be

[17] American Medical Association, Council on Foods and Nutrition: *J. A. M. A.* 146:35, 1951; Roy, W. R., and Russell, H. E.: *Food Industries* 20:1764, 1948.

[18] Huggart, R. L., *et al.: J. Am. Dietet. A.* 30:682, 1954.

the best sources of vitamin C in a study of the various canned fruits and vegetables by Pressley and associates.[19]

Questions and Answers on Vitamin C

A brief summary of the clinical significance of vitamin C is reprinted by kind permission of the Florida Citrus Research Foundation, Lakeland, Florida:

Is a slight vitamin C deficiency important clinically?
Dallyn and Moschette [20] note that "the lack of ascorbic acid in the diet may not be great enough to cause actual scurvy, but a *slight deficiency can cause minor changes in the body which are too important to neglect*."

How common is infantile scurvy?
Evidence obtained at Johns Hopkins University [21] in autopsy studies of 1126 infants under one year of age shows that scorbutic lesions existed in the bones in nearly 6% of infants—10 times as many as were diagnosed clinically.

How do citrus fruits help in weight reduction?
Three ways: (1) to minimize appetite when eaten one-half hour or one hour before meals, (2) to combat hypoglycemia (low blood sugar) between meals, and (3) to maintain ample vitamin C intake.[22]

How high a vitamin C intake is needed to correct a deficiency?

[19] Pressley, A., *et al.*: *J. Nutrition* 28:107, 1944.

[20] Dallyn, M. H., and Moschette, D. S.: *J. Am. Dietet. A.* 28:718, 1952.

[21] Follis, R. H., Jr., *et al.*: *Bull. Johns Hopkins Hosp.* 87:569, 1950.

[22] Joliffe, N., and Alpert, E.: *Postgrad. Med.* 9:106, 1951.

Up to ten times the normal requirement,[23, 24, 25] and if the deficiency is of long duration it is recommended that such an increased daily intake be continued for a year or longer.[23]

Why is natural vitamin C superior to synthetic?
The simultaneous intake of the many other nutritional factors may promote greater utilization of the vitamin C in natural sources. Indeed, natural sources of the antiscorbutic vitamin, notably the juices of citrus fruits, may prove to be more efficient and complete in their action.

Will high citrus intake help prevent spontaneous abortion?
Javert [26] finds that it will. By means of a comprehensive regimen including high citrus intake (350 mg. vitamin C daily) plus additional synthetic vitamin C and vitamin K, he obtained live deliveries in 88.1% of 134 pregnancies in patients with a previous record of only 4.8%.

Do adolescents get enough vitamin C?
They frequently hit "rock bottom" because too often their lunches are of the hot-dog, soft-drink, candy-bar type.[27] In a study of 2500 teen-agers from all types of families, Mack [28] found that only 50.3% of boys and 52.4% of girls obtained recommended daily allowances of vitamin C in their daily food intake.

Why is vitamin C important for the surgical patient?

[23] Gale, E. T. and Thewlis, M. W.: *Geriatrics* 8:80, 1953.

[24] Joliffe, N.: *J. A. M. A.* 129:613, 1945.

[25] Tisdall, F. F., and Joliffe, N.: in: *Clinical Nutrition,* edited by Norman Joliffe, *et al.,* New York, Paul B. Hoeber, 1950, pp. 586-601.

[26] Javert, C. T.: *Obst. & Gynec.* 3:420, 1954.

[27] Young, Charlotte M., *et al.: J. Am. Dietet. A.* 27:289, 1951.

[28] Mack, Pauline Beery: through *Food Field Reporter* 21:48, Apr. 20, 1953.

Principally for wound healing and for resistance to infection. Schilling and associates describe vitamin C as the most important single substance in promoting fibrosis and collagen formation, and they state that "large amounts of vitamin C are nontoxic and seem indicated in all cases of major surgery."

Why do elderly patients need citrus fruits?
Principally to maintain a high level of vitamin C intake which "may avert a vascular crisis" and "operate to restore tissue and capillary lesions." The inositol content also affords significant lipotropic activity.[29]

Why are citrus fruits important in treatment of acne?
On a diet devoid of vitamin C five out of ten subjects showed a "very pronounced exacerbation" of the acne that was present in a mild form at the start of the test,[30] and Morris[31] has reported excellent results with high citrus intake in the management of acne vulgaris.

Are infants allergic to orange juice?
Joslin and Bradley[32] found no instances of gastrointestinal disturbances due to orange juice, and less than 2% of 406 infants and children reacted to skin tests. By keeping peel oil at a minimum in orange juice, even this low incidence of sensitivity is reduced by another two-thirds.

Is there any danger of toxicity from high intakes of vitamin C?

[29] Krehl, W. A. and Cogwill, G. R.: *Food Research* 15:179, 1950.

[30] British Medical Research Council, Food Factors Committee, *et al.*: Vitamin C Requirement of Human Adults, London, England, *Medical Research Council Special Report* Ser.-2-No. 280, HMSO, 1953.

[31] Morris, G. E.: *Am. Pract. & Digest Treat.* 5:658, 1954; and *Postgrad. Med.* 14:443, 1953; and *A.M.A. Arch. Derm. & Syph.* 70:363, 1954.

[32] Joslin, C. L., and Bradley, J. E.: *J. Pediat.* 39:325, 1951.

No toxic effects have ever been demonstrated. Lowry [33] administered 1000 mg. daily to four adults for a period of three months with no ill effects, and in a larger group of elderly patients Cass and his associates administered 4000 mg. daily for three months with no evidence of toxicity.

What is the clinical value of the citrus snack?

It is recommended by Mack [34] as an easy means of greatly increasing the vitamin C intake of teen-agers who obtain a large part of their total food intake by between-meals nibbling. The universal availability and popular taste appeal of citrus products make the "Citrus Snack" a favorite with patients of any age once its nutritional significance is understood.

Lemon Remedies

The following is a partial list of lemon remedies which appeared in the book *Encyclopedia of Health and Home* by Drs. Wood and Ruddock.[35]

Asthma: Many cases of asthma have been relieved by taking a half tablespoon of the juice of a lemon before each meal and upon retiring.

Cold and coughs: Roasted lemon, when properly prepared, is one of the most effective remedies for coughs and colds. Following are the directions for its use: It should be roasted or baked in a moderately heated oven for about half an hour, or until it begins to crack open or the juice begins to exude . . . Dose, from one-half to a tablespoonful of the juice, sweetened to the taste before each

[33] Lowry, O. H., *et al.: Proc. Soc. Exper. Biol. & Med.* 80:361, 1952.

[34] Mack, P. B.: at Conference on Research in Medicine, Florida Citrus Commission, Lakeland, 1954.

[35] Chicago: Vitalogy Assoc., 1921.

meal and again before retiring at night. In severe cases, take it every three or four hours.

Corns: Lemon applied to corns a few times is an efficient remedy. Bind on the corn and leave on overnight.

Felon: Cut off the end of the lemon and insert the finger which has the felon in the lemon and bind it on. In the morning the matter will be drawn almost to the surface when it can be removed . . . When taken in time it will scatter the felon.

Headache: To the juice of two large lemons add one quart of common table tea, made from the best green tea. Add the juice to the tea when the latter is boiling hot, and when cool bottle for use. Dose, one teacupful, repeated in two or three hours.

Heartburn: One dose of half tablespoonful, diluted with a little water, is usually sufficient for a cure.

Removing stains from the hands: Use clear lemon juice; it will remove many kinds of stains from the hands.

Seasickness: Anyone liable to an attack of seasickness . . . can easily prevent the seasickness by sucking a lemon as soon as the sick feeling begins. It will pass away almost immediately.

Warts: Steep in vinegar the inner rind of a lemon for twenty-four hours, and apply it to the wart. The lemon must not remain on more than three hours, and should be applied fresh every day.

Whooping Cough: The following remedy has never been known to fail in relieving whooping cough in four or five days, if given when the child first whoops. Take one lemon and slice thin; add half a pint of flaxseed, two ounces of honey and one quart of water: simmer, but do not boil, four hours; when cool strain and if there is less than a pint of the mixture, add sufficient water to make a pint.

Dose, one tablespoonful four times a day, and in addition, a dose after each severe fit of coughing.

Lemon Juice as a Beauty Aid

Washing the face every night with the juice of a lemon and allowing it to remain on until morning is said to gradually remove tan, freckles or blackheads. Another method claimed effective for removing freckles is taken from an old recipe book:

One ounce of lemon juice, a quarter of a dram of powdered borax, and half a dram of sugar; mix in a bottle, and allow to stand a few days, when the liquor should be rubbed occasionally on the hands and face.

Lemon juice rubbed into the scalp before shampooing is considered effective in eliminating dandruff. A lemon-milk preparation is employed for whitening and softening the skin of the hands and face. Just enough milk is poured over a slice of lemon to cover it. This is allowed to stand for two hours. It is then strained and after the hands and face have been washed, the prepared solution is applied and allowed to dry.

Because of its astringent action, lemon juice is rubbed over wrinkles as an aid in eliminating them. The juice is left to dry on the skin and later removed with olive oil.

The following appeared in the *Herbalist Almanac*, 1964: [86]

The lemon is an all-around beauty aid. Lemon juice makes a nice rinse for the hair. It will remove the soap film much better than plain water. Use the strained juice of one lemon in two quarts of water or double the amount.

[86] Hammond, Ind.: Indiana Botanic Gardens.

A slice or section of lemon can be used on the hands and finger tips after washing them with soap. Stains can be removed from the fingers with a slice of lemon dipped in peroxide.

For a delightful skin lotion, make a mixture of 1 oz. of strained lemon juice, 3 oz. of rose water, and 1 oz. of glycerine. Use this soothing lotion every day for the face and hands.

Other Uses of the Lemon

A few drops of lemon juice sprinkled over sliced bananas, apples or avocados will prevent them from turning brown for a considerable period of time. Frequent applications of lemon juice is said to remove ink, rust or mildew stains from cloth. For this purpose, some recipes call for the addition of milk or salt to the lemon juice. In using the salt, a paste is made with the juice and then applied to the rust stains on the fabric. The mixture is left on for half an hour or more, then the cloth is rinsed in water and hung out in the sun to dry.

XII

the herb of the cherokees

*. . . even as the green herb have I given you all
things.—Gen. 9:3.*

PRIOR TO 1830, the Cherokee Indians occupied the upper
valley of the Tennessee River. They were friendly to the
English in the wars against the French, and ceded lands
to Governor Glen in 1755 for the construction of forts
within their territory. They rendered valuable service to
the army of General Jackson against the British, and as
early as 1817 their lands were ceded to the United States
in exchange for lands on the Arkansas and White Rivers.
During the Civil War, the Cherokees sided with the
Confederates, and took part in the Battle of Pea Ridge.
Later, however, they became divided into two factions.

The Cherokees were regarded as the most progressive
of the Indian tribes. Within one year they were trans-
formed into a literate nation through the efforts of their
chief, Sequoya. Very little is known of Sequoya's early life;
however, when he was about 48 years of age he con-
ceived the idea of inventing an alphabet so that his people
could read and write in their own language. He began this
great work in 1809, and by 1821 he had succeeded in

constructing an alphabet that was so perfect and easy to use that within a few months most Cherokees could read and write. It is of interest to note that Sequoya had never known any other language. Printing characters were cast in Boston in 1827, and the publication of the first Cherokee newspaper soon followed. Later, books were also published.

Golden Seal

Indian tribes of North America relied almost entirely on the plant kingdom for their medicinal needs. One of the favorite herbs of the Cherokees was golden seal. This is a small perennial plant with a thick, fleshy yellow rhizome, and produces a solitary rose-colored or whitish flower. The fruit somewhat resembles the raspberry but is not edible.

This plant grows in moist, rich woodlands in various parts of the United States, but more abundantly in the North Eastern sections. The name golden seal was given to the herb because of the seal-like scars on the golden-yellow root. In botany it is known as *Hydrastis canadensis*.

Golden seal was used by the Cherokees as a remedy for sore mouth, inflamed eyes, and as a bitter tonic in stomach and liver disorders. They also employed it externally for diseases of the skin, and their remedies soon became very popular among the early pioneers and settlers. The fresh root is quite juicy and was highly valued by the Indians as a dye for their garments and a stain for their faces.

Medical History of Golden Seal

The first medical reference to golden seal appeared in Barton's *Collections for a Vegetable Materia Medica* (1798), in which he credits the Cherokee Indians with the introduction of the plant to the settlers. In the third part of this work (1804), Baron mentions that in Western Pennsylvania an infusion of golden seal root in cold water was used as a wash for inflammation of the eyes. He also remarked that "it supplies us with one of the most brilliant yellow colors with which we are acquainted."

Hand (*House Surgeon*, 1820) also referred to the plant and stated that, "It may be given in form of powder or strong tea made by boiling, in indigestion, the secondary stages of low fevers and in all cases of weakness in general."

Rafinesque, in his *Medical Flora of the United States* (1828), defined the yellow alkaloid of golden seal as a "peculiar principle *hydrastine* of a yellow color." He devoted considerable attention to the plant, and stated that, "Internally it is used as a bitter tonic in infusion or tincture in disorders of the stomach, liver, etc." He mentioned that it was employed by the Indians for many external complaints, adding that some of them also prepared an infusion for internal use as a diuretic.

Other doctors began employing the herb in their practice and wrote enthusiastic accounts of its value. The *Thomsonian Recorder* of 1833 reviewed the medical properties of golden seal described by others, and added:

> The importance of this article . . . for the relief and removal of bowel complaints in children should be extensively known. It is not only a corrector of the stomach, a regulator of the bowels, and a vermifuge for children, but it is an admirable remedy for the peculiar sickness attendant on females during their periods of utero-gestation, called morning sickness. It admirably relieves stomach oppression, nausea, and heartburn.

Professor John King issued his first edition of *The Eclectic Dispensatory of the United States of America*

(1852), in which the medicinal use of hydrastis (golden seal) was given a most careful review. Many of the virtues ascribed to the plant by early writers were omitted as being overrated. The re-evaluation of the herb, its properties, uses and preparations were then carefully discussed in this work, and the remedies brought before the attention of the Eclectic branch of the medical profession. In consequence of its general adoption by the Eclectics, a great demand for golden seal was created and the plant became an article of commerce. Hydrastis was declared an official drug in the pharmacopoeia of the United States in 1860.

Early Uses in Skin Diseases

Although the yellow color of golden seal root was fully appreciated by the Indians, their enthusiasm for this virtue of the herb was not shared by the medical profession. Its medicinal employment was objectionable as the powdered root stained everything with which it came in contact, and was extremely difficult to remove. This problem, however, was overcome by the investigations of Professor Bartholow who demonstrated that hydrastis could be combined to form hydrastine hydrochlorate and be free of staining.

According to Dr. John V. Shoemaker, this preparation was successfully employed in skin diseases. In many instances, however, a fluid extract of golden seal was taken internally in conjunction with the external use of hydrastine hydrochlorate. Numerous case histories in which this treatment was favorably employed were cited by Dr. Shoemaker in the book *Drugs and Medicines of North America*.[1] A few typical examples are given as follows:

The good results so far realized from the topical

[1] J. U. Lloyd & C. G. Lloyd (Cincinnati: Robert Clarke & Co. 1884).

application of hydrastine hydrochlorate may be illustrated by the following cases in which it has been employed in the clinical services of the Philadelphia Hospital for Skin Diseases.

Acne. Patient age 17. Forehead, cheeks and chin covered with small red papules associated with black points—acne punctata—and papulo pustules, digestion feeble, bowels torpid. Ten drop doses of the fluid extract of hydrastis were given three times daily before meals and the face was sponged night and morning with an aqueous solution of hydrastine hydrochlorate containing ten grains of the salt to the ounce. In ten days the patient showed signs of improvement, and in six weeks after being placed under treatment he was discharged cured.

Eczema of the face. Patient age 3. Scalp and face covered with thick crusts, which upon removal exposed red raw and infiltrated patches, digestion poor, constipation at times followed with diarrhea. Half a drop increased to a drop of the fluid extract of hydrastis was administered in milk three times daily with the effect, in course of twelve days, of improving the child's general condition and lessening somewhat the local inflammation. The red and infiltrated patches remained stubborn, notwithstanding the use of the ordinary ointments. At the end of the second week of the constitutional treatment, one ounce of lard with twenty grains of hydrastine hydrochlorate was used freely over the parts. The red and thickened patches gradually disappeared and in two weeks time from the beginning of the topical application only a slightly desquamating (scaling off) surface remained.

Eczema of the ears. Patient age 27. The right and left ears were red, somewhat thickened and covered with scales. The skin back of each pinna was in a similar condition with several fissures at their connection with the side of the head. The inflammation of the ears had originally been excited by a dye, and had resisted the usual local remedies. The ointment of hydrastine hydrochlorate, of the same strength as mentioned in the previous case, was used with good effect within six days. The ears in about three weeks had acquired their natural size. The fissures healed quickly, and when last seen, about ten days ago, only a little roughness of the integument was apparent.

Golden Seal in the 20th Century

Many popular modern preparations for the eyes, such as eye drops, eye washes, etc., include hydrastine as one of the ingredients. In the book *Back To Eden*,[2] the noted American herbalist, Jethro Kloss, cites the use of golden seal in morning sickness, sore mouth and eyes, eczema, indigestion, catarrh, etc.

Dr. William Fox, M.D., employed it in his practice as a stimulating tonic, claiming that "it has a powerful action upon the mucous membranes, which renders it useful in cases of gastric debility, indigestion," etc. He further states that "it also possesses considerable influence on the nervous system and in combination with *capsicum* is a remedy in chronic alcoholism; for this purpose and also as a general tonic in indigestion we use equal parts of the tincture of *hydrastis, cayenne,* and *chelone glabra.* Dose: 25 to 30 drops in two tablespoonfuls of water, three times a day before meals. Omitting the cayenne it is a good tonic for weakly children, in doses of from 5 to 10 drops in sweetened water according to age."

Drs. Wood and Ruddock cited golden seal as a remedy in various disorders. They especially valued it in the treatment of "some forms of dyspepsia" and recommended the decoction in the dose of "one tablespoonful 3 times a day; of the tincture, one to 2 teaspoonfuls 3 times a day."

Dr. Swinburne Clymer devotes considerable attention to the value of the herb in *Nature's Healing Agents.* Here are a few excerpts:

[2] Longview Publishing House, Coalmont, Tennessee, 1964.

It improves the appetite and assists digestion. In the weak and debilitated stomach, especially where there are nervous disturbances or if the gastric membrane be clogged with congested or catarrhal mucus, and in cases of gastric ulceration, *Hydrastis* given in small and frequent doses generally will give relief both to the gastric membrane and to the nervous system.

Hydrastis (golden seal) may be made to act specially upon the stomach, bronchi, urinary aparata or genitalia by its combination with agents that especially influence any one of these several departments. With agents like *Aralia, Prunus,* or *Comfrey,* it gives tone and vigor to the respiratory organs . . .

In combination with bicarbonate of soda it is an excellent wash for . . . children's sore mouth and also other forms of sores in the mouth and of the gums.

Locally, the influence of *hydrastis* is very superior to most other agents. In erysipelas, sore throat, leucorrhea, eczema, . . . it is excellent. In these washes it should be combined with:

> Tinct. Hydrastis   1 oz.
> Tinct. Myrrh   ½ oz.
> Tinct. Echinacea   ½ oz.

This is a non-poisonous, non-irritating antiseptic, healing and soothing agent and may be applied as frequently as required.

Potter's New Cyclopaedia of Botanical Drugs and Preparations gives the following information on golden seal:

Tonic, laxative, alterative, detergent. Since about 1847 Golden Seal has figured conspicuously in the botanic practice. The name was given to this plant by Thomsonians, who employed the root. The demand for "concentrations" was the means of discovering the two alkaloids contained in this drug—Hydrastine, the white, and Berberine, the yellow—

besides others of less value. For many years these and the powdered root were the chief forms administered. Latterly, however, the drug in the form of a fluid extract is the most used and popular. It is a very valuable remedy in disordered states of the digestive apparatus. As a general bitter tonic it is applicable to debilitated conditions of mucous tissues. As a remedy for various gastric disorders it takes a leading place, acting very beneficially in acute inflammatory conditions. It will be found of value in all cases of dyspepsia, biliousness, and debility of the system. It is especially indicated in catarrhal states of the mucous membranes, gastric irritability, ... Externally it is used as a lotion ... and as a general cleansing application.

XIII

the intriguing herb that hides
from man

*. . . they traded in thy market wheat of Min-
nith, and Pan-nag, and honey, and oil, and balm.*
— *Ezek. 27:17.*

ASIATIC GINSENG, BOTANICALLY known as *Panax schin-
seng,* is found in the Orient, while the American Ginseng
called *Panax quinquefolium* or *Five Fingers Root* is a native of the United States. Ginseng has very peculiar traits.
It loves seclusion and hides from man as though it possessed some type of reasoning intelligence, seeking unfre-
quented deep shaded forests and hillsides for its home. It
passes many years dormant in the ground, and keeps a
record of its age on the stem of its root. It is one of the
slowest growing plants known. Wild ginseng is never
found near stagnant water and experiments have shown
that if the plant is forced to use such water it becomes
sick. It also shuns low, wet ground with insufficient drain-
age. Sometimes, however, it is found very close to running
water. At one time it was believed that ginseng could not
be cultivated, but today we find that it is successfully
grown in many parts of the world.

More About the "Man-Plant"

The Chinese composed the name *ginseng* from two words meaning "man-plant." Quite often the roots bear a remarkable resemblance to the shape and form of a man, sometimes in all detail. For over 5000 years, 400 million Chinese, each of many generations, have steadfastly maintained that ginseng had great merit as a remedy in a variety of ills. It would be foolish to suppose that for 50 centuries the Chinese were basing their faith in ginseng on nothing but sheer superstition. Ginseng would have been discarded by the Chinese long ago if it did not produce genuine results.

At one time, the prize of possessing the countryside in which ginseng grew caused bitter fighting between the Chinese and Tartars. In order to protect his precious supply, one Tartar king is said to have built a wooden palisade around an entire province.

In the early days, ginseng root was considered the property of the Chinese emperor. It was required of those gathering the root that two and ⅔ pounds be given free to the monarch. He paid an equal weight in silver for any collection in excess of that amount, which was actually only about a quarter of its market value.

Aphrodisiac, Reactivator and Rejuvenator

The Chinese declare that the sick take ginseng to recover their health, while the healthy use it to resist disease and make themselves stronger. The men over forty all use ginseng to preserve their virile powers and completely avoid the male climacteric so common among Westerners at this age. In escaping this decline, they are also able to retain their virility as long as they live and it is common in China among men who use ginseng to procreate children at the age of 60, 70, or over.

The ancient medical book of India, *The Atherva Veda,* states that ginseng aids in bringing forth "seed that is poured into the female that forsooth is the way to bring forth a son. . . . The strength of the horse, the mule, the goat and the ram, moreover, the strength of the bull [ginseng] bestows on him. . . . This herb will make thee so full of lusty strength that thou shalt, when thou art excited, exhale heat as a thing on fire."

The action of ginseng in this respect is not considered merely as an aphrodisiac which acts as a stimulant but instead is claimed to be a reactivator and rejuvenator of the gonads and the organism as a whole. The organism depends upon the hormones poured into the blood stream by the gonads for its vitality.

Sir Edwin Arnold, author of *The Light of Asia,* states:

> According to the Chinese, Asiatic Ginseng is the best and most potent of all Cordials, Stimulants, Tonics, Stomachics, Cardiacs, Febrifuges, and above all, will best renovate and invigorate failing forces. It fills the heart with hilarity, while its occasional use will, it is said, add a decade to human life. Have all these millions of Orientals, all these many generations of men who boiled Ginseng in silver kettles and praised heaven for its many benefits, been totally deceived? Was the world ever quite mistaken when half of it believed in something never puffed, never advertised, and not yet fallen to the fate of a trust, Combine or Corner?

Invigorates and Prolongs Life

The earliest Chinese book on the medicinal value of herbs was written by Emperor Shen-ung, about 3000 B.C. Ginseng is regarded as the highest, most potent among thousands of herbs mentioned in this work. Shen-ung who is referred to as the Father of Agriculture and Medicine, claimed that ginseng was "a tonic to the five viscera, quieting the animal spirits, strengthening the soul, allaying fear, expelling evil effluvia, brightening the eyes, opening the heart, benefiting the understanding and if taken for some time, it will invigorate the body and prolong life."

In 1274 A.D. when Marco Polo traveled through China, he found ginseng in general use. He made a study of it and if he had felt that it was of no importance, he would not have bothered to mention it in the record of his journey.

The Chinese use the root faithfully if they can afford it, as a disease preventative. Sucking the juice of the root, or preparing it as a tea is considered a definite requirement after hard work or "indulgences." Wounded soldiers on the battlefields are given ginseng to strengthen them while being carried to army hospitals.

Grows in Radioactive Soil

Because it is more potent and more difficult to secure, the wild ginseng sells for a much higher price than does the cultivated. It is believed that the rejuvenating action of ginseng on the sex glands is due to certain radioactive substances that it absorbs from the soil. Being of organic origin, these radioactive substances are beneficial rather than harmful and are *unlike* the strontium 90 and other *inorganic* fallout products. It is assumed that the wild plant is more potent because it selects its own location and chooses the ones where the radioactivity of the soil is highest.

Many stories of the Far East claim that ginseng hunters wait until dark before searching for the plant because the flower emits a phosphorescent glow. It is said that the flowers are so sensitive that at the slightest sound they will immediately fold up and their glow can no longer be seen. For this reason the hunters shoot arrows at these "lights" and in the morning when they find the arrows, they dig up the plant. It is possible that this phosphorescence of the ginseng flowers is related to the high radioactive content of the plant.

A Panacea of All Disease?

From a publication *New Scientific Discoveries in Regeneration,* we find the following information:

> The latest discovery from China is ginseng, the rejuvenation herb, considered by the Chinese as a panacea of all diseases. It is believed by its enthusiasts that ginseng overcomes disease by building up general vitality and resistance and especially by strengthening the endocrine glands, which control all basic physiological processes, including the metabolism of minerals and vitamins. Chinese ginseng-users consider as infantile Western attempts at rejuvenation by monkey gland operations. Centuries of experience among millions of people have convinced them that in ginseng exists a natural method of rejuvenation, of restoring vitality to depleted glandular organs by feeding them the mysterious radioactive elements that ginseng has proven to contain.

Father Jartoux, a missionary in China in the early part of the 18th century witnessed the gathering and use of ginseng. An early American account of Father Jartoux's experiences is given in part:

> While on a journey among the mountains of Tartary, Father Jartoux met in various instances with the plant, and with the people employed in collecting it. He states that the root is found principally in thick forests, upon the declivities of mountains, the banks of torrents, and about the roots of trees. It never grows in the open plains or valleys, but always in dark shady situations, remote from the sun's rays.

In the dark woodland, the soil would be enriched by decaying leaves dropped by trees whose roots sink deep into the subsoil and absorb the radioactive substances not found in the top soil of open land.

A mandarin in Father Jartoux's company noticed on one occasion that the Good Father was so exhausted that he was no longer able to sit on horseback, and gave him a ginseng root. Father Jartoux took only half of it and within an hour his fatigue was completely gone. He stated that he was in perfect agreement with the Chinese belief that the Fountain of Youth is contained within ginseng. He described the herb as being a physiological invigorant, a rejuvenator, and also believed that it prolonged life. "The Chinese," he said, "use a decoction of the root, for which they employ about a fifth part of an ounce at a time. This they boil in a covered vessel with two successive portions of water, in order to extract all its virtues." Father Jartoux also wrote:

Discovery in North America

The report of the high value of ginseng at Pekin led to an inquiry among Europeans, as to whether the plant was not to be found in parallel latitudes, in the forests of North America. Father Lafiteau, a Jesuit missionary among the Indians, after much searching, found a plant in Canada answering the description, and sent it to France. In 1718 M. Sarrasin published in the Memoirs of the Academy an account of the American ginseng, which, together with one published by Lafiteau the same year seemed to put its identity with the Chinese vegetable beyond a doubt.

In Canada, the French soon began exporting the herb to the Far East. In the forests of the United States the search for wild ginseng was launched, and the export of the herb became a profitable business. In 1784, George Washington wrote: "In passing over the mountains, I met a number of persons and pack horses going in with ginseng." Large amounts of ginseng were taken to China by American ship owners who came back stocked with teas, silks and spices. Gunn wrote in 1834: "It is found in great plenty among the hills and mountains of Tennessee and brought to Knoxville daily for sale."

More Precious Than Gold

Ginseng is considered so valuable by the Chinese that at one time the Mandarin or Imperial Ginseng sold for $200 an ounce or $3,200 a pound! Sometimes authorities would present a distinguished person who would be in serious need of ginseng, with an ounce or two. The government set up depots for the storage of the herb which were heavily guarded by strong military forces. During various periods in Chinese history, the export of ginseng was considered a capital crime!

Why this herb, so highly regarded by the oldest civilization in the world should be almost entirely ignored by the West appears to be somewhat of a mystery. Scarcely any scientific research has been done on it, consequently little is known or even heard about it. The Russians, however, have been devoting an enormous amount of attention to the ginseng plant. An investigation of the herb by Russian scientists prior to World War II was conducted by the Institute of Experimental Medicine of the U.S.S.R. The purpose was to discover whether the remarkable properties ascribed to ginseng by the Chinese was due to its radioactive contents. It was learned that the so-called *taiga* variety of wild ginseng could be grown only in radioactive soil. It was in the wildest parts of the Sikhote-Alni mountain range, where this type of wild ginseng was found to flourish. Several Russian experimental stations were placed in this area. Soviet investigators proved that the roots contained many radioactive properties including the ability to emit warmth. The roots had to be kept in lead paper wrapping to prevent the escape of their radioactive emanations and to preserve their remarkable virtues. When the second World War began, these investigations were interrupted.

Research Kept Secret

For some reason the report of this particular research was kept secret and never revealed to the scientific world. We can well imagine just how important the results of this investigation must have been, when some years later in the early part of the Korean War, a report stated: "Russians grab entire Korean supply of Ginseng, valued at $120,000,000." Referring to the Russian research of Asiatic Ginseng, C. S. Ogolevec, in his *Cyclopedia Dictionary of Medical Botany* 1955, says:

> During the Korean War millions of dollars of Korean Ginseng was sent to the U S S R. when the northern armies overran Korea. The Soviet scientists investigated the properties of this Ginseng and found that many of the things the Orientals were saying about Ginseng were true. They gave its structure as $C_{32}H_{36}O_{19}H_{41}O_8$, stating among other properties that it strengthens the heart, and the nervous system and increases the hormones, etc. It contains Panaxin, Panaquilom, Schingenin, etc.

It has recently been learned that the Russians have now planted in the Maritime Province of South Siberia, tremendous plantations of ginseng, costing many millions of rubles!

Some decades ago, a Russian electrobiologist, Professor Gurwitch, made an announcement to the scientific world that a peculiar type of ultra-violet radiation called *mitogenetic* radiations were found to be emitted by onions. These radiations had the property of stimulating cell growth and activity. It was found that cell proliferation was stimulated when the mitogenetic rays of the growing center of one onion were allowed to impinge on the growing center of another. Garlic and ginseng were found to emit the same radiations and these radiations seemed to have a rejuvenating effect.

Results of American Reserach

The eminent American physiologist, Dr. G. W. Crile, has made a special study of the mitogenetic radiations which are given off by the human body which were similar to those of ginseng. It is apparent, then, that through the mitogenetic radiations, ginseng acts as a general physiological revitalizer, giving off a species of radioactive rays with which it inwardly irradiates the system.

A study of ginseng as a source of Gurwitch mitogenetic radiations was made by Professor Lakhovsky, an eminent Russian biologist residing in Paris. He has found that ginseng, particularly the Wild Manchurian ginseng, emits an ultra-violet type of mitogenetic radiation that has a beneficial effect on the sexual and other endocrine glands. When these glands are stimulated, they increase hormone-producing activity. He believes that the increase of these various hormones is responsible for the rejuvenating effects claimed by the Chinese physicians, and accepts these claims as scientifically valid

P. M. Kourenoff, in his book *Oriental Health Remedies*, writes:

Asked by the author which of the Chinese-Tibetan remedies he considered best for the treatment of sexual impotence, the late Dr. S. N. Chernych of San Francisco stated, "Ginseng! Oriental healers are successfully curing patients of sexual impotence by the use of ginseng, and sexual impotence is one of the most difficult disorders. I can state from personal experience, that the Oriental physicians have cured several men whom I and several other doctors tried to help."

War Veterans Restored to Health

The author can verify this from his own personal observation in the city of Harbin, Manchuria, during the years 1920-1923. Harbin was crowded with civilian refugees and interned units of the Russian National (White) Army. Most of these ex-soldiers had served in the First World War, and later in the Civil War. Nerve-shattered and ill, many of these veterans were suddenly stricken with sexual impotence.

They stormed the offices of regular doctors of medicine, and receiving no help, finally turned to the Chinese healers. It is reported that all of them were cured by the Chinese practitioners, chiefly with the aid of ginseng, occasionally supplemented by, or combined with, other substances. Three of six persons known to the author were completely cured by the use of ginseng alone.

When all else has failed to restore sexual vigor, ginseng can be counted on, if there is any hope at all. There is nothing mysterious or supernatural about its curative properties. No one need fear its use if directions are followed carefully. We should think no more of taking a dose of ginseng for sexual impotence than taking a dose of castor oil for constipation, for ginseng is as much a vegetable as the castor bean.

Several Varieties Available

Several varieties of ginseng are known to medicine, not all of equal virtue. The best is the Wild Manchurian ginseng which grows only in the Sikhote-Alin Mountains of Eastern Manchuria and in the Maritime Province of Siberia. The cost of this particular variety of ginseng often skyrockets to several thousand dollars for a single root during a period of shortage.

Many remedies for sexual impotence are not only impractical but even harmful, because they have but one effect, to stimulate sexual vigor. Ginseng, on the contrary, rejuvenates the entire system. Any man drinking the ginseng infusion as instructed, five or six winters in succession, will feel considerably younger than his years in every way. Also, those who once restore sexual vigor with ginseng rarely if ever experience impotence again. Of course, the normal vigor of a man reduces naturally with his advancing years, and this must be taken into consideration. No one who has ever lived in China could fail to notice the sanguine faces of the wealthy Chinese. This is explained chiefly by the fact that all the well-to-do Chinese regularly drink ginseng infusion.

How Ginseng Rejuvenates

When the famous English vegetarian, Thomas Parr (who lived past the age of 150) accepted the invitation to dine with the king of England, he died following the eating of meat. John Harvey, the discoverer of the circulation of blood, dissected the body of Thomas Parr and found that his gonads were as powerful and large as those of a young man. This indicates that the strength of the gonads is related to longevity for it is an accepted fact that the endocrine glands are basically responsible for the general vitality and organic functioning of the body and determines its potency, youthfulness, health, and longevity. In youth, the gonads are strong, powerful and active. A gradual decline becomes evident with the advancing years and in old age the gonads finally become atrophied. In rebuilding these cells by the use of ginseng, they are made to regain the characteristic of youth. Consequently they flood the system with a new supply of life-giving hormones by which process the body becomes rejuvenated.

It is universally agreed by those who have used ginseng over a considerable period of time that the root defintely does have a strengthening effect upon the gonads although this rebuilding action is a slow and gradual one.

For Maximum Benefits

Various authorities assert that it is necessary for genuine regeneration of the gonads that the new sexual energy which ginseng imparts be conserved and not wasted.

We are told that the seminal lecithin and sex hormones are both present in the seminal fluid. These must be conserved during the period when ginseng is taken so that they may be reabsorbed into the bloodstream for the purpose of rejuvenation and not lost through sexual indulgence. When this newly created energy is reabsorbed, it is then transmuted into increased vitality of the brain and entire body. This is the real goal. For maximum benefits, then, we are advised that the use of ginseng should be accompanied by a period of continence.

Further Medical Use of Ginseng

Among the learned physicians of China as well as the Chinese public itself is the general belief that ginseng is a universal medicine. It is possible that the action of ginseng on the endocrine glands gives the body the power to make better use of the vitamins and minerals, and in this way helps to overcome nutritional deficiences.

The Greeks referred to Ginseng as "the plant of the sorcerers" and believed that it possessed magical virtues. In Japan, ginseng is considered a longevity herb. Among the North American Indians it was employed as a remedy for stomach disorders, sore gums, menses, and was sometimes used as a love potion.

One of the earliest accounts of ginseng in America was give by Samuel Henry in his *American Medical Family*

Herbal. He mentions the herb as valuable in "weakness from excess of venery, pain in the bones after colds, and gravally complaints." The dry root grated in water is mentioned in Bowher's *The Indian Vegetable Family Instructor*, 1836, as a remedy for gas in the stomach. A very popular guide of the old days was *Gunn's Family Physician* which referred to ginseng as follows: "It is useful in nervous debility, weak digestion and feeble appetite, and as a stomachic and restorative. It is considered a very valuable medicine for children and has been recommended in asthma, palsy, and nervous affections generally."

An official report from a former United States Consul at Seoul, Korea, states:

> From personal experience and observation I am assured that Korean Ginseng is an active, and strongly healing medicine. Western people appear to regard the virtues of Ginseng claimed by Orientals rather contemptuously—as imaginary or based on superstition. The evidence is that the mystical value attached itself to Ginseng after its virtues had been practically ascertained. (U.S. Consular Report, No. 65)

A Modern Medical Opinion

Although ginseng has been almost completely ignored by Western medical men of modern times, one physician was open-minded enough to give the root a careful clinical study in his medical practice. This man was A. R. Harding, M.D., of Columbus, Ohio. He found that in various ailments from which his patients suffered, they recovered more quickly when given ginseng than any other form of medicine or treatment. Dr. Harding gave up his medical practice and spent the rest of his life studying the fascinating herb. He grew the plant himself, became an authority on its cultivation, and wrote a book called *Gin-*

seng and Other Medicinal Plants.[1] This book is largely devoted to ginseng culture; however, Dr. Harding included a chapter of his experiences regarding the medicinal value of ginseng. A few excerpts from this chapter are quoted as follows:

For several years past I have been experimenting with Ginseng as a medical agent and of late I have prescribed, or rather added it, to the treatment of some cases of rheumatism. I remember one instance in particular of a middle-aged man who had gone the rounds of the neighborhood doctors and failed of relief, when he employed me. After treating him for several weeks and failing to entirely relieve him, more especially the distress in bowels and back, I concluded to add Ginseng to his treatment. After using the medicine he returned, saying the last bottle had served him so well that he wanted it filled with the same medicine as before. I attribute the curative powers of Ginseng in rheumatism to stimulating to healthy action of the gastric-juices; causing a healthy flow of the digestive fluids of the stomach, thereby neutralizing the extra secretion of acid that is carried to the nervous membranes of the body and joints, causing the inflammatory condition incident to rheumatism.

Ginseng combined with the juices of a good ripe pineapple is par excellent as a treatment for indigestion. It stimulates the healthy secretion of pepsin, thereby insuring good digestion without incurring the habit of taking pepsin or after-dinner pills to relieve the fullness and distress so common to the American people.

It would take too long an article for me to enumerate the cases that I have cured; but I think it will suffice to say that I have cured every case where I have used it with one exception and that was a case of consumption in its last stages; but the lady and

[1] A. R. Harding Publishing Co., Columbus, Ohio.

her husband both told me that it was the only medicine that she took during her illness that did her any good. The good it did her was by loosening her cough; she could give one cough and expectorate from the lungs without any exertion.

A neighbor lady had been treated by two different physicians for a year for a chronic cough. I gave her some Ginseng and told her to make a tea of it at meal times and between meals; in two weeks I saw her and she told me that she was cured and that she never took any medicine that did her so much good, saying that it acted as a mild cathartic and made her feel good. She keeps Ginseng in her house now all the time and takes a dose or two when she does not feel well.

Various Methods of Using Ginseng

Dr. Harding mentions that at a meeting of the Michigan Ginseng Association, Dr. H. S. McMaster presented a paper on the uses of the plant, which appeared in the *Michigan Farmer*. The methods of preparing ginseng were suggested as follows:

1. The simplest preparation and one formerly used to some extent by the pioneers of our forest lands, is to dig, wash and eat the green root, or to pluck and chew the green leaves.

To get the best effect, like any other medicine, it should be taken regularly, from three to six times a day and in medicinal quantities. In using the green root we would suggest as a dose a piece not larger than one to two inches of a lead pencil, and of green leaves one to three leaflets. These, however, would be pleasanter and better taken in infusion with a little milk and sweetened and used as a warm drink as other teas are.

2. The next simplest form of use is the dried root, carried in the pocket, and a portion as large as a kernel of corn, well chewed, may be taken every two

or three hours. Good results come from this mode of using, and it is well known that the Chinese use much of the root in this way.

3. Make a tincture of the dried root, or leaves. The dried root should be grated fine, then the root, fibre or leaves, separately or together, may be put into a fruit jar and barely covered with equal parts of alcohol and water. If the Ginseng swells, add a little more alcohol and water to keep it covered. Screw top on to keep from evaporating. Macerate in this way 10 to 14 days, strain off and press all fluid out, and you have a tincture of Ginseng. The dose would be 10 to 15 drops for adults.

Put an ounce of this tincture in a six-ounce vial, fill the vial with a simple elixir obtained from any drugstore, and you have an elixir of Ginseng, a pleasant medicine to take. The dose is one teaspoonful three or four times a day.

The tincture may be combined with the extracted juice of a ripe pineapple for digestion, or combined with other remedies for rheumatism or other maladies.

4. Lastly I will mention Ginseng tea, made from the dry leaves or blossom umbels. After the berries are gathered, select the brightest, cleanest leaves from mature plants. Dry them slowly about the kitchen stove in thick bunches, turning and mixing them until quite dry, then put away in paper sacks.

Tea from these leaves is steeped as you would ordinary teas, and may be used with cream and sugar. It is excellent for nervous indigestion.

These home preparations are efficacious in neuralgia, rheumatism, gout, irritation of bronchi or lungs from cold, gastroenteric indigestion, . . . and other nervous affections, and is especially adapted to the treatment of young children as well as the aged. Ginseng is hypnotic, producing sleep, an anodyne, stimulant, nerve tonic, and slightly laxative.

(*Reference:* Dr. Raymond Bernard (A.B., M.A., Ph.D.), *Herbal Elixirs of Life,* Health Research, Mokelumne Hill, California, 1959.)

XIV

the secret of perpetual youth

*Who satisfieth thy mouth with good things; so
that thy youth is renewed like the eagle's:*
—*Psalms 103:5.*

Fo-ti-Tieng

A HIGHLY POTENT variety of *Hydrocotyle asiatica* known
as *Hydrocotyle asiatica minor,* is also called Fo-ti-Tieng.
It is found only in certain jungle districts of the Eastern
Tropics. Professor Menier of Paris studied the herb and
claimed to have found in it an unknown vitamin which he
termed vitamin X. This vitamin appears to have a marvelous rejuvenating effect on the brain cells and endocrine
glands.

Lived for 256 Years

Fo-ti-Tieng gained its popularity due to the fact that
the renown Chinese Herbalist, Li Chung Yun, who lived
to be 256 years of age, used the herb daily. This aroused
the interest of the French Government and led to the es-
tablishment of an experimental station in Algeria where a

committee of experts could study the plant. A research foundation in connection with a college in Colombo, Ceylon, received an endowment from the English Government for the same purpose.

Professor Li Chung Yun was born in 1677, and in 1933 the *New York Times* announced the death of this remarkable Oriental whose life span had reached over two and a half centuries! His age was officially recorded by the Chinese Government and confirmed by the investigations of Professor Wu Chung Chich, head of the Chang-Tu University. The correctness of Li's amazing age was also borne out by the fact that he had outlived 23 wives and was living with the 24th at the time of his death.

A Youthful Appearance

Professor Li gave a course of 28 lectures on longevity at a Chinese university. At the time he gave this course of three-hour-long lectures, he was over the age of 200. Those who saw him declared that he did not appear older than a man of 52; that he stood straight and strong, and had his own natural hair and teeth.

An article printed in the Toronto *Globe* regarding Li Chung Yun is given in part as follows:

A professor in the Minkuo University claims to have found records showing that Li was born in 1677, and that on his 150th and 200th birthdays, he had been congratulated by the Chinese government— as well he might. Men who are old today declare that their great-grandfathers, as boys, knew Li as a grown man

Dieticians should look into this. It is unlikely that during the first 100 years or so of his life Li Chung Yun knew anything about vitamins or calories; and certainly no radio instructions about setting up exercises awakened him at the dawn. Early in life—

either about 1690, 1750 or thereabouts—this Chinese lad developed a penchant for collecting herbs . . . And here is the point. What did Li discover? Some neglected weed that contained the elixir of life?

Rejuvenating Herbs

The article mentions that Li advised that it was the part of wisdom to "keep a quiet heart, sit like a tortoise, walk sprightly like a pigeon, and sleep like a dog." Commenting on this, the article states:

> But that is merely camouflage. There are many people without number today who have the tortoise temperament and whom it is almost impossible to awaken in the morning, but they pass on without any notice in cable dispatches. "Walking sprightly like a pigeon," is among the arts lost by man, and it may be that the loss of his favorite herb led to Li's untimely taking off; which is a discouraging conclusion to the life story of a calm Oriental who watched the centuries come and go.

It is claimed that Li Chung Yun's longevity was due to his strictly vegetarian diet, his calm and serene attitude toward life, and the fact that he regularly used two powerful rejuvenating herbs prepared as teas. One of the herbs was Fo-ti-Tieng and the other was ginseng. With the exception of ginseng *root*, Li would eat only the food that is produced *above* the ground.

A special research on the herb Fo-ti-Tieng was conducted by P. de Layman, M.H.P.A., director of the Herbal Institute of London. He wrote an article which appeared in several British publications as well as the American Magazine, *Health Culture*. The article was entiled, "A Remarkable Plant from the Far East," and is given as follows:

The "Elixir of Life"

Arriving next month at the London docks from the Eastern tropics is the largest consignment yet to reach England of what must surely be one of the most intriguing and valuable cargoes that has ever been introduced to Western medical science. Packed in several double canvas bales, marked only with a number for secrecy, is the result of several weeks of careful collecting and drying of a low-growing herb found only in certain jungle districts in the Eastern tropics, known to Chinese medicine as Fo-ti-Tieng, the "Elixir of Life" or "Long Life Elixir." The event of this shipment, consigned to the Herbal Research Institute, recalls the considerable interest aroused in the world's press when in 1933 there died near Pekin Professor Li Chung Yun at the age of 256—the oldest man so far as records show. The fact that he was married 24 times rather goes to bear out the correctness of his attributed age. During his life he was a sort of botanic chemist or herbalist who regularly made himself an infusion or tea from an herb which he found in his earliest years and thenceforth used throughout his extraordinarily long and active existence. This herb is Fo-ti-Tieng, known to botanists as Hydrocotyle Asiatica Minor—not to be confused with the ordinary taller plant, Hydrocotyle Asiatica, as has happened mostly in America. Fo-ti-Tieng is not a plant that would attract attention of ordinary folk, yet it has been renowned among Chinese and Eastern Indian scholars as a food possessing great life-sustaining properties. It was Professor Li Chung Yun, however, whose lectures on Fo-ti-Tieng and the way to healthy longevity first began to attract the attention of other than native students and introduced the plant to certain European doctors resident in Pekin.

The Search for Vitamin X

After clinical tests had been made over an extensive

period, its rejuvenating virtues made such an impression that the French Government, hearing of it, procured living plants and succeeded in establishing a plantation and experimental station in Algeria; and later even the usually less enterprising British Government, gave a grant of land and money to the Ayurvedic College of Research, of Colombo, Ceylon, for the purpose of furthering the study of this unique herb. A French biochemist, Jules Lepine, conducted an examination of the herb and found that the leaves and seeds yield a rare tonic property, probably an alkaloid, which has a marked energizing effect on nerves and brain cells; but what seems the more exciting news resulting from an analysis carried out by Professor Menier, of the Academic Scientifique, near Paris, and experts in Algeria—both independently—is the discovery of what certainly appears to be a new vitamin not known in any other food or herb.

This he described as the "youth vitamin X," which property is, in the opinion of all authorities interested in Fo-ti-Tieng, that chief and peculiar virtue of the plant which exerts a rejuvenating influence upon the ductless glands, the healthy functioning of which, as most readers may know, are the means by which the brain and body are maintained in healthy activity. An interesting sidelight is thrown upon the unique vitamin aspect by the assertion many years ago of Nanddo Narian, a then 107 years old Indian sage, to the effect that Fo-ti-Tieng provides a missing ingredient in a man's diet without which he can never wholly control disease and decay.

The Finest Herb Tonic

As a research herbalist, I have given long and close attention to Fo-ti-Tieng, and have found it in practice to be the finest of all herbal tonics and nutrients. It appears to have no equal in the treatment of general debility and decline. Digestion is strengthened, other foods better absorbed and the process of metabolism increased, with a noticeable improvement in the appearance of the patient. I find it best administered in powder form, and this is certainly more handy too. In larger doses it proves to be a safe aphrodisiac, when required.

As for this remarkable plant promoting long life—who knows? I have every reason to think that it does so. Our antique friend, Professor Yun and other old men and women of the East seemed to do great justice to the herb's reputation. Perhaps the name "Elixir of Life" given it by the Chinese may be somewhat exaggerated, if immortality is implied; still, there can be little doubt that the regular use of Fo-ti-Tieng can assure for us the next best thing—a useful, ripe old age.

Gotu Kola

Gotu Kola grows in India, the Islands of the Indian Ocean, and in some parts of Southern Africa, and is believed to contain remarkable rejuvenating properties similar to those of Fo-ti-Tieng and Ginseng. The natives of India use the plant medicinally as a diuretic or stimulant to the kidneys and bladder as well as a blood purifier and alternative. Many years ago a French physician residing in the Island of Mauritius claimed that the herb had merit in the treatment of leprosy.

The following interesting article appeared in the *Ceylon Daily News*, Dec. 22, 1932, entitled "Gotu Kola—The Secret of Perpetual Youth":

The Power of Staying Young

Man's dream has always been to discover the secret of perpetual youth, and many men have devoted all their lives to this problem. We have heard of Ponce de Leon who sought restoration of youth from the waters of a charmed fountain in Florida, the Kintan of the Chinese, the Red Elixir of Geber and the Vital

Essence of Augsburg. The Bolivian Indians made an elixir out of a thornless cactus which, it is said, had the power of keeping men young right up to their death, while not so long ago a Swiss named Spalinger claimed to have found a serum that prolonged life to 150 years.

Instead of believing that the secret of perpetual youth could be thus obtained, they should have tracked an elephant in the woods of Ceylon and observed what the behemoth ate for his lunch. Ten chances to one it would have been Gotu Kola. Had they done this, the world would be growing this life-giving plant as commonly as lettuce and there might not be on earth today anyone with a body that could truthfully be termed senile.

Gotu Kola has every ancient history behind it. It was known to writers of India hundreds of years ago, always as a longevity plant. It is a small herb that creeps along the ground, having fan-shaped leaves of a pale green color. The taste is slightly pungent, but eaten with rice or bread it is delicious. It is claimed that this vegetable will increase the vitality of 70 and 80 to that of 40. The leaves have a marked energizing effect on the cells of the brain, and can preserve it indefinitely. The leaves are not a stimulant but a brain food.

Strengthens and Revitalizes

A German scientist, Baron Gogern, tells us that a wild elephant, in captivity at Deshapur, was once rejuvenated and bore a calf after Gotu Kola was sent for and mixed in her diet. A few of the leaves eaten raw every day will strengthen and revitalize worn out bodies and brains to a remarkable degree and will prevent brain fag and nervous breakdown.

In cases of mental troubles, blood pressure, abcesses and rheumatism, the efficacy of Gotu Kola has been highly valued. In elephantiasis, bruises, swollen parts and rheumatic swellings, the oil of the herb or the juice extracted from it will check fever associated with these affections. The powder of the herb, taken by drying in the sun, is sprinkled on ulcers with effective results. For mental weakness and memory improvement, the powder of the leaves, in small doses, is given.

To realize the truth of these assertions, it is only necessary to look back a few hundred years into the medical history of the East. "Two leaves a day will keep old age away." This is the claim made by the Sinhalese for Gotu Kola, this famous longevity plant which grows profusely in Ceylon. In India, the leaves are extensively used by religious orders to develop spiritual power and to prolong the existence of the brain.

Food for Mental Power

Miss Mary E. Forbes of America, the tutor of Her Highness, the widowed Queen of Mandi State in the Punjab, in 1914, commenced eating it in her salads, and after a few months she never knew what brain fatigue was, and felt so physically well that she could not find enough to do to use up her energy.

It is the belief of the Sinhalese and the Indians also that only one or two of the leaves of this herb are necessary daily to bring about a gradual return to health and strength, provided the body is exposed to the sun. If this is eaten daily, it is said that disorders like rheumatism, neuritis and nervous breakdown can be banished entirely from the constitution and would be an important factor in breeding a better race. It is claimed that Gotu Kola will increase the span of life by 50 years by developing a brain incapable of breaking down for a very long time.

It is a well known fact that no skeleton or corpse of an elephant has ever been found that died a natural death. The villagers of Ceylon assert that they keep their youth and strength for hundreds of years because they eat Gotu Kola.

Live to Be 100-Plus

Not only is it certain that the average span of human life could be considerably increased if people ate Gotu Kola, but it will also be a fact that the proportion of human beings who die a natural death will be very small. It will mean that monkey glands will be given the go-by for this new herb, which makes grandpa act like his grandson and puts a girlish smile on the wrinkled face of grandma.

To be informed that such remarkable herbs exist in the plant kingdom is nothing short of a major revelation. Unfortunately mankind as a whole is so rooted in the belief that the life span can reach only an average of 60 or 70 years that they fail to see the profound truth, that this so-called "standard" is *not normal* at all. Consequently such information is dismissed as being highly exaggerated or ridiculous and there the matter ends. Yet everyone will readily admit that there are wonderful instances of longevity in the animal world. Crocodiles and tortoises for example, live for centuries. If such things are possible in the ordinary course of nature in the animal world, why should we doubt the ability of God to produce even greater results in His highest creation, which is man?

If it can be proven that one human being has lived past the age of 100, 200 or even 300 years, it would certainly be sufficient evidence that a universal principle of longevity exists. It then follows that *anyone* may use this principle. We have seen that Li Chung Yun bore witness to the truth of this universal law, but he was by no means the only one.

Other Instances of Longevity

The examples of longevity are too numerous to be detailed even in a book devoted solely to this subject; how-

ever, a few examples may be cited here. Haller, the celebrated English physician, during his time collected more
than one thousand cases of persons in Europe who attained the ages of from 100 to 170 years. In Baker's
Curse of England a list of 100 individuals is given whose
ages ranged from 95 to 370! Thirty of these exceeded
120 years of age, while 22 reached a life span of 150 upwards. Modern statisticts cite examples of persons in the
United States as well as other parts of the world who
have attained the age of 100 and over.

If we turn to the Bible we find many examples of extremely advanced age are set before us in such persons as
Adam, Methuselah, Noah, Enoch, etc. Time and again,
attempts have been made to discredit such Biblical accounts of longevity by saying that they were only symbol-
ical or that the calendar in ancient days was all out of
proportion to our present measurement of time. That
such Biblical records also have hidden spiritual meanings
cannot be denied, but to explain away such things as
being *only* symbolic, without actual manifestation in the
world of time and space, is to admit of unbelief in the
power of God to operate on the plane of nature. How can
anyone hold such an erroneous opinion in the light of the
fact that God has created nature? On the other hand,
those holding the opinion that the ancient calendar was
grossly out of line with our present measurement of time
will find it exceedingly difficult to explain away the age of
an individual such as Li Chung Yun, whose birth was recorded in *modern times* and whose death consequently
was publicized in many newspapers throughout the world.

Again, some people argue that though they believe the
Biblical records of longevity, they also believe that they
occurred only through special Divine Dispensations to a
select few, and were not intended for the average man.
Assurance not only of the principle of longevity, but that
it was intended for everyone, is clearly stated in Scripture
as Promises, provided we work with God's laws instead of

against them: *There shall be no more thence an infant of days, nor an old man that hath not filled his days: for the child shall die an hundred years old.—Isa. 65:20.* In other words, death at the age of 100 would be considered so premature as to resemble that of an infant! And, . . . *for as the days of a tree are the days of my people, and mine elect shall long enjoy the work of their hands.—Isa. 65:22.* (The "elect" are those who follow God's ways and His laws.) Here the normal standard of age is compared to a tree which lives for centuries. And again, *His flesh shall be fresher than a child's: he shall return to the days of his youth:—Job 33:25.* Here is a promise that it is never too late to reform.

Views of Science on Longevity

Science tells us that the cells of the human body can never become old. Every minute, millions of cells are becoming inert and are discharged through perspiration, the urine, feces, etc., and new ones are being formed. Within a period of two years, ninety percent of all the cells are renewed, and not a single cell of the eye is more than a few years old. It should be remembered that during this process which continues throughout life, nature is adding young new cells, not aged cells.

As an experiment, Dr. Alexis Carrel of the Rockefeller Institute, kept a piece of chicken heart alive for 34 years. He concluded that, "Tissue cells are essentially immortal. Give cells all the essential nutrition they need, remove promptly all wastes and poisons and they can be kept alive indefinitely." He ended his experiment when nothing new could be learned by continuing it.

Dr. William Kinnear wrote:

We cannot defy death. But we may by searching find certain secrets of nature, and apply them to the renewal of the organs whose decay is constantly go-

ing on in the body . . . Without nutrition there is no
repair of the body. Hence, G. H. Lewes states, that
"if the repair were always identical with the waste,
life would only then be terminated by accident, never
by old age."

In the opinion of O. Phelps Brown, M.D.:

> If the body develops itself slowly and healthfully,
> as it always will in its natural state, it is only rea-
> sonable to suppose that the periods of infancy, child-
> hood, and adolescence or maturity would be greatly
> prolonged, by the more simple conformity to the
> original laws of our own being; the period of youth
> might and would be extended to what we now call
> "old age"—say three score and ten, and "three score
> and ten" would be but the beginning of the vigorous
> manhood to be indefinitely prolonged, reaching on to
> a hundred or even two hundred years. The true
> philosophy of life is to live and enjoy—to use and
> not abuse the essentials to human longevity and hap-
> piness. As we read in Holy Writ, in the earlier history
> of man, when the air was free from infection, the soil
> exempt from pollution, and man's food was plain and
> natural, individuals lived, on the average, four or five
> hundred years.

In 1948, Dr. Thomas B. Gardner announced that in
experimenting with fruit flies he had increased their life
span by forty-five percent. He fortified their diets with the
B vitamins, pantothenic acid, pyridoxine, and yeast nu-
cleic acid. He commented, "This clearly shows you can
add years to your life and slow the process of aging."

Dr. Henry Sherman of Columbia University conducted
an intensive study of diet and longevity. Experimenting
with rats, Dr. Sherman and his associates doubled the
amount of vitamin A in the diets of one group of rats
while the other group received the usual adequate diet
which had kept them healthy and thriving all their lives.

The male rats given the increased amount of vitamin A lived five percent longer (for the males) and ten percent longer (for the females) than the group fed on the regular diet.

Vitamin A was again doubled and the rats getting the quadruple amount every day lived ten percent longer (for males) and twelve percent longer (for the females) than the other group. It was observed that the extra years of life enjoyed by the rats were *not senile years*. When the amounts of vitamin A were again doubled, there was no further extension of their life span.

The recommended daily minimum requirement of vitamin A for the adult man or woman is 5,000 International Units. It may be possible that 20,000 units would result in better health and longer, useful lives. Until experiments have been conducted on human beings, no one can know for sure.

Dr. Thompson, in his *Medical Dictionary*, says, "At some future day there can be little doubt that the value and duration of life will be greatly extended beyond what it is at present; greatly beyond what we can at present imagine."

(*Reference:* Dr. Raymond Bernard (A.B., M. A., Ph.D.), *Herbal Elixirs of Life,* Health Research, Mokelumne Hill, California, 1959)

XV

herbs that condition and beautify the hair

I beheld till the thrones were cast down, and the Ancient of days did sit, whose garment was white as snow, and the hair of his head like the pure wool.—Dan. 7:9.

HERBS HAVE BEEN used for thousands of years for conditioning and beautifying the hair. Many famous and beautiful women of the past developed their own herbal hair formulas and guarded these secrets jealously.

Philippine natives steep a few slices of aloe blades in cold water, and this preparation is used on the hair as a tonic. This is also highly valued as a hair conditioner by the natives of Java and Malaya. The Balinese, noted for their shimmering black hair, condition it by washing with herbal preparations, concluding with the application of coconut oil to which has been added the aromatic fragrance of ylang-ylang flowers.

Saffron was used by the ladies of the court during the reign of Henry VIII to give a reddish tone to their hair. As this herb was extremely expensive, those who could not afford its virtues used the yellow marigold flowers as a substitute.

An old herbal states: "An infusion of mullein leaves was used by the Roman ladies to tinge their tresses of the golden colour so much admired in Italy: and now in Germany a wash made from mullein flowers is highly valued." Centuries later, it was a popular custom for Italian ladies to expose their hair to the noonday sun, wetting it with aromatic vinegars, and allowing the sun to dry it. This process was repeated several times.

In certain Oriental countries, the use of herbal hair dyes seems to be almost universal. In Persia, the hair remains black from childhood to old age, due to the use of such dyes.

Herbal Hair Recipes

The herbal recipes given in this chapter are not original. As previously stated, such recipes have been used both in the past and present by many people throughout the world who attest to their efficiency in adding life, beauty, tone, or color to the hair. Perhaps among these, you may discover a favorite of your own.

HERBAL SHAMPOOS

For Normal Hair

1. Fill a container with water and bring to a boil. When the water boils, add a heaping teaspoonful of each of the following herbs: nettle, sage, maiden hair, southernwood, and peach leaves. Allow to simmer for 15 to 20 minutes. Strain, and add shavings of castile soap while the liquid is still warm enough to dissolve them.

2. Another method is to place one cup of camomile blossoms in one quart of water. Simmer for 10 minutes. Strain, and add one ounce of castile soap shavings.

For Oily Hair

1. This recipe is used for oily light hair. The superfluous oil is absorbed by sprinkling the hair thoroughly with powdered orris. After 5 or 10 minutes, this powder may be brushed out. When applied in the evening, it may be left on during the night, and brushed out in the morning. A dry shampoo may also be used to advantage by anyone suffering from a cold, or for any reason where a wet shampoo is inadvisable.

2. For black or brown hair which appears greasy or lifeless: Boil ¼ ounce of southernwood, ¼ ounce of rosemary, and ¼ ounce of quassia chips in enough water to make a wash, and allow to simmer for 10 minutes. Strain, and add castile soap shavings.

AROMATIC VINEGARS

1. To one quart of white vinegar, add ½ ounce of each of the following herbs: rosemary, marjoram, and lavender flowers, with just a pinch of ground cloves. Allow to steep for a week or ten days, then strain through a fine cloth. Proportions may be changed according to your own desire. You may also add to this recipe, cut orris root and/or calamus.

2. A very fine or delicately scented vinegar may be made with the fresh flowers of roses, clove-pink, and orange, or the dried flowers of lavender or elder. If more strength is desired, oils may be added to the vinegar which has been steeped with herbs. Two or three drops of the essential oils of rosemary, bergamot, lavender, etc., to one quart of the prepared vinegar is generally sufficient. You may select your own aromatic herbs and oils. Many beautiful women in the past created wonderful recipes by blending together various botanicals of their own choice.

These had the added attraction of being uniquely individualized, dressing up the personality as well as the hair.

DYES AND RINSES

Hair must be shampooed before applying dyes or rinses. A test is always made to ascertain the absorbing characteristics of the hair before using hair dyes. This may be done by snipping off a small lock of the hair and using it for a test.

Henna as a hair dye or rinse has been recognized for ages. A new attractiveness can be added to faded brown hair, or auburn types of hair, by the use of a henna rinse. Other herbs may be incorporated to obtain different shades. For example, the effects of henna can be darkened by the addition of cloves, while indigo added to henna results in shades of deep brown. A deeper red can be obtained by the addition of logwood chips. As a hair dye, henna paste is made with the powdered herb. It is also used on darker types of hair which require more than just a rinse. Remove rinse with a shampoo before getting a permanent.

Dye for Lovely Hair of Golden Brown

Steep one handful of garden sage in one pint of water for several hours. Put two rounded teaspoonfuls of powdered henna and one teaspoonful of ground cloves into a dry bowl and mix together. Pour a little of the sage tea over this mixture to make a thin paste, and keep stirring until smooth.

After you have shampooed and rinsed your hair, partially dry it, then cover it thoroughly with the paste mixture. Tie a cloth around the head, and leave the paste on for about 30 minutes; longer if a darker shade is desired. Remove the cloth and rinse the hair with warm water to remove the paste. This recipe is purported to give the hair a beautiful shade of reddish-brown with golden highlights.

Persian Method of Dyeing the Hair

The Persians use the following method of dyeing the hair. The hair is shampooed first to remove the oil, then some henna powder is mixed with warm water until it attains the consistency of a paste, and is applied to the hair. The paste is left on the hair for more than an hour and is then washed off with warm water. With this application, the hair attains a dark orange or saffron color. The powdered leaves of the indigo plant are now made into a paste in the same manner, and applied to the hair. The indigo paste is allowed to remain on the hair for an hour and a quarter, and is then washed off. The process is now complete. The dark hue appears several hours later through the oxidation of the indigo, and is purported to make the hair a jet black.

If the Persians prefer to color the hair a chestnut brown rather than black, they mix one part of henna and three parts of powdered indigo leaves. This is applied to the hair after it has been shampooed. The longer the paste is allowed to remain on the hair, the darker the shade becomes. Usually, one hour is considered sufficient to produce a light brown color, and an hour and a half for dark brown. If the first dyeing is too light, the paste is renewed.

Henna Rinse

Add ½ ounce of henna (less for lighter shades of hair) to one quart of boiling water, and steep for 20 minutes. Strain after cooling if cut leaves are used. Hold the head over a basin and pour the liquid over the hair. Repeat this process, by using the liquid caught in the basin, until the desired shade is obtained. Darker types of hair require more rinsing than lighter types. The rinse is followed with clear water.

Sage Rinse

To darken and bring out the highlights of brunette and darker types of hair, a sage rinse is considered effective. To one quart of boiling water, add a handful of sage. Steep for about 30 minutes. The longer the sage steeps, the darker the color becomes. After steeping, strain and allow to cool. Hold the head over a basin and pour the sage rinse over the hair. Dip a brush in the rinse and quickly part the hair, brushing the rinse all over the head. Pour the balance of the rinse over the hair, using a second container to catch the liquid so that this process may be repeated several times. The hair is then dried.

Rinse for Blond Hair

To bring out the highlights of blond hair, add three or four tablespoonfuls of camomile flowers to a pint of water. Boil slowly from 20 to 30 minutes and strain when cool. Hair must be free from soil, so it is necessary to shampoo first before using the rinse. While holding the head over a basin, pour the decoction over the hair. Dip a brush in the rinse caught by the basin, and work the liquid into the hair by parting the hair and brushing. Pour the remaining liquid over the hair several times and repeat the brushing. Do *not* use a clear rinse after the camomile rinse if you wish to retain the sweet smelling fragrance of this aromatic herb.

Rinse for Faded Blond Hair

1. The following recipe helps to keep blond hair from turning a "mousey" shade. It cleanses the scalp and keeps it free of loose dandruff, and brings a glistening sparkle to

the hair. Mix ¼ ounce of quassia chips and ¼ ounce of camomile flowers in enough boiling water to make an adequate rinse. Simmer for 10 or 15 minutes, then strain. Apply once or twice a week.

2. A favorite recipe of the English beauties was to use a mild henna rinse followed by a camomile rinse. This was purported to give a beautiful sheen to auburn and blond hair.

Rinse to Enliven Dull Dark Hair

1. Make a mixture of the following: ¼ ounce of southernwood, ¼ ounce of rosemary, and ¼ ounce of quassia chips. Boil together in a sufficient amount of water for approximately 10 minutes, and use as a rinse when cool. This recipe helps to bring out the natural color of the hair.

2. Dr. Fernie, early in the century, wrote that an ounce of rosemary steeped in boiling water and allowed to stand until cold makes one of the best hair washes known to enliven the color of the hair. More modern ideas include the use of a small amount of borax added to this wash. Sometimes elder flowers are combined with rosemary.

3. Maiden hair fern or yarrow were popular English rinses.

For Grey or Falling Hair

1. From a recipe book printed in 1880 we find: "The hair may be prevented, generally for a considerable time, from turning grey, by keeping the head cool and by using occasionally, sage tea with a little borax added. With a small sponge apply to every part of the head just before the time of dressing the hair."

2. The American Indians used a simple remedy for grey or falling hair. In the spring, they cut off the end

branch of the common grape vine and tied a bottle or gourd to it so that the sap could be collected. The sap was used as a lotion and rubbed freely into the scalp and roots of the hair. The Indians often used an alternate method by making a tea of the roots of the grape vine and employing it as a wash. This was used two or three times a month whenever they first observed a tendency for their hair to become grey or start falling. Once the problem was under control, the wash was used only once a month as a preventative.

3. To darken hair that is turning grey, the following method is used: Mix one pint of strong sage tea to one pint of bay rum, and one or two ounces, more or less, of glycerin, depending upon the natural oil of the hair. Shake this mixture thoroughly and rub well into the roots of the hair, using a small amount each night. This should be continued every night until the desired results are obtained.

4. Cut up one ounce of tag alder bark and steep in two quarts of water; allow to boil down to one quart. This is employed as a final rinse whenever the hair is washed. It is claimed that its use will gradually color white or grey hair, giving it a very natural and beautiful shade of brown.

5. The following recipe is taken from an old medical herbal:

> Wash the head once a day with warm strong sage tea. It will promptly check the falling out of the hair. If the use of this be continued for a sufficient length of time it will make the hair thick and strong.

6. When used as a rinse or wash, gobernedora, rosemary, nettle, or peach leaves are reputed to check falling hair.

7. For stimulating the growth of the hair, an old herbal suggests the use of a nettle-vinegar preparation. A

strong decoction (resembling the color of coffee) is made by adding plenty of fresh dry nettles to equal proportions of water and vinegar. This decoction is rubbed gently into the scalp once a day. Each morning, the scalp is washed with cold water.

HAIR CONDITIONERS

1. The inner bark of the wild cherry tree boiled over a low flame for 20 minutes and used as a wash when strained and cooled, is considered a very good hair conditioner. Excellent results have been reported after 30 days' use. Ragwood is also claimed to be very beneficial when used as a rinse after shampooing.

2. Put one chopped parsnip root and ½ teaspoonful of parsnip seeds in ¼ cup of olive oil. Boil for 5 minutes, strain and rub into the scalp and hair. This solution restores the gloss to the hair and is reputed to stimulate the growth.

3. Put a handful of nettle into one quart of water and boil slowly for two hours. Strain when cool and bottle for use, applying to the scalp every other night. This must be prepared fresh every few days, as it will not keep for a prolonged period of time. Its use will make the hair soft and glossy.

4. Another recipe advises: "Dip the hairbrush in a little nettle tea each morning and brush the hair vigorously for 5 minutes."

5. Very fine hair will attain considerable body by the use of a nettle rinse. Prepare as an infusion, a good handful of nettle to one quart of water. Strain and use. If the hair is put up in curlers directly following this rinse, it will, when dried, comb out into a fluffy head of hair. A few drops of rosemary oil may be rubbed over the hair to give it a beautiful sheen.

To Curl or Set the Hair

1. The following is taken from a recipe book printed in 1846. Iceland moss is soaked in cold water from one to two hours. It is then drained and dissolved in boiling water. Powdered gum arabic can be used for the same purpose when dissolved in water. "It is used by the ladies to make their hair curl firmly, and remain in any desired position. It is applied by moistening the comb in the solution and passing it through the hair."

2. Put two pints of soft or rain water into a double boiler. Add one teaspoonful of quince seed and two tablespoonfuls of flaxseed and boil until the volume is reduced to half. Strain through a cloth and use. It may be scented if desired by adding either oil of rosemary, almond oil, etc.

3. A rinse of rosemary is reputed to be a great aid in preventing the hair from uncurling when subjected to a damp atmosphere.

Brushing Out Snarls

Drying long or curly hair with a towel often produces snarls that are painful to comb or brush out. The snarls untangle more easily if oil of rosemary is applied to your hairbrush just as you are ready to use it.

Pour a teaspoonful of oil of rosemary into the palm of the hand, and then work it lightly into your hairbrush. The excessive oil remaining on the hand can be rubbed over the damp hair. Brushing can now be done without the usual painful tugging. If you have extra thick hair, it would be wise to add an extra teaspoonful of the oil, as the hair will tolerate a good amount. Don't let the strong spicy aroma of this oil discourage you from trying the suggested amount, for though its fragrance at first appears quite potent it gradually fades and is completely unnoticeable within a few short hours.

The virtues of the oil of rosemary extend beyond its ability to untangle snarls, as it is an excellent conditioner for both the hair and scalp, and leaves no trace of oiliness once the hair has been fully dried.

TO STRAIGHTEN KINKY HAIR

One ounce of alkanet root is added to 1 pound of vaseline and boiled for 1 hour, then strained through a flannel cloth. After the mixture has cooled, ¼ ounce of tincture of benzoin and a few drops each of oil of Bergamot and oil of Citronella is added. This preparation is applied with the finger tips to the roots of the hair, morning and night.

DANDRUFF

1. A tea prepared from the leaves and bark of the willow tree is said to be effective in eliminating dandruff. The solution is rubbed well into the scalp.
2. ½ cup of mint leaves, ½ cup of vinegar, one cup of water; boil together slowly for 5 minutes. Strain and rub well into the scalp.
3. A nettle rinse is a favorite with many people as a means of eliminating dandruff.

Note: When preparing any of the herbal hair recipes given in this chapter be sure to keep the containers covered in which decoctions are boiling or infusions are steeping.

(References: *The Herbalist Almanac*, and *Botanical Catalog*, Indiana Botanic Gardens, Hammond, Indiana.)

XVI

miscellaneous herbs

*And the earth brought forth grass, and herb
yielding seed after his kind, and the tree yielding
fruit, whose seed was in itself, after his kind:
and God saw that it was good.—Gen. 1:12.*

IT WOULD NOT be possible to devote a full chapter to
every plant or plant food which has shown medicinal activity or exceptional nutritive merit. To do so would require many volumes. However, a few more botanicals
may be briefly cited, and these are given in alphabetical
order as follows:

ALFALFA
(Medicago sativa)
Synonyms: Buffalo herb, Lucerne.

Alfalfa is a legume as peas and beans are. However,
the leaves, sprouts and seeds are eaten, rather than just
the seeds alone. It is one of nature's oldest legumes, and
is known to have been cultivated for over 2000 years.
The Arabs, centuries ago, used it as a feed for their
horses and claimed that it made the animals swift and

strong. They decided to try it themselves and became convinced that its use was so beneficial to the health and strength of the human body that they named the "grass" *Al-Fal-Fa,* meaning Father of All Foods.

Today, alfalfa stands as one of the largest leaf crops in the world. In the United States alone, 16 million acres are devoted to its cultivation. This clover-like perennial plant is often productive from 10 to 15 years or more.

Alfalfa, a Deep-Rooted Legume

Scientists have suggested that deep-rooted or deep-feeding plants may become particularly valuable sources of food for man and animal. Most plant foods are shallow surface feeders whose roots do not penetrate much further than the soil is cultivated and fertilized. Alfalfa possesses deep feeder roots which burrow far into the earth seeking out minerals in the deep subsoil which are inaccessible to other plants. During the first three weeks of growth (under normal conditions), the young roots of alfalfa are known to make ten times more root growth than the stem!

A former Secretary of the Department of Agriculture for the State of Kansas once wrote:

> The root (alfalfa) in its development is most interesting for its great power of penetrating, under at all favorable conditions, to the very bowels of the earth. Many instances are on record of roots having been dug up or otherwise exposed, some of which showed a length and penetration of 38 feet, while even greater depths of 50 to 66 feet and more are recorded.

Valuable Properties Contained in Alfalfa

Vitamins. Many years ago, oats were considered solely as horse feed, yet today the nutritive value of oatmeal is well-recognized. At present, alfalfa is still commonly thought of merely as a food for livestock; however, scientists are discovering that it possesses substances which are valuable to the health of human beings. It contains vitamins A, E, K, B^6, D and U. A deficiency of vitamin A in the body may result in a condition known as night blindness. Vitamin E is believed by some authorities to be very important to the health of the heart, muscles, and sex glands. As a healing agent in peptic ulcers, scientists believe that vitamin U shows great promise, as it prevents ulcers in laboratory animals. Vitamin U is also present in cabbage juice, and is thought to be the factor responsible for the remarkable cures of stomach ulcers in human patients reported by Garnett Cheney, M.D., of the Department of Medicine of Stanford University. Vitamin K helps to clot the blood properly and protect against hemorrhages. This vitamin has also been found effective in preventing and curing high blood pressure in test animals and may eventually turn out to be more important to the health of man than is presently known. (Alfalfa is extremely rich in vitamin K—most plants possess very little.)

Other Properties: Alfalfa is very high in protein and also contains phosphorus, iron, potassium, chlorine, sodium, silicon, magnesium, and trace elements. It is particularly rich in calcium which may be obtained in almost pure form by reducing the leaves to ashes. Science tells us that calcium is essential for the proper development and health of the bones and teeth. Calcium, phosphorus, and iron all work together in keeping the teeth in strong condition. On this point, Dr. Sherman Davies, of the University of Indiana, said: "The use of alfalfa as food for humans would be a great boon, and those who produce it will be doing the world a vast service in saving the teeth of all ages."

The muscles also require calcium, and medical men have reported that quite often people who have suffered chronically from cramps in the legs and feet obtain relief almost immediately once they begin to use enough calcium. The heart, too, is a muscle and needs calcium to regulate the rhythm of the heart beat. Laboratory solution in which hearts are placed and kept alive outside the body is largely composed of calcium.

The protein content of alfalfa is exceptionally high—18.9 percent as compared with 16.5 percent in beef, 3.3 percent in milk, and 13.1 percent in eggs. The muscles of the body are composed of protein, and a lack of it causes the muscles to break down, resulting in fatigue and weakness. Flabby muscles in the intestines and stomach may result in constipation, as they cannot contract and expand properly in order to move the food along the digestive tract. Poor posture may often result from lack of protein. The hair, skin and nails are also made of protein, and cannot replace dead tissues if they are not supplied with this important substance.

Alfalfa also contains eight known enzymes. Enzymes are promoters of chemical reactions necessary to enable foods to be assimilated in the body.

Care in Growing Alfalfa for Human Use

Alfalfa which is grown for human use is cultivated and handled with great care. Fields are kept free from weeds and foreign plants. Useless stems are separated from the leaves, and the plant cured and dried in the best possible way to preserve as much of the vitamins and other elements as possible.

Alfalfa Tea

Some botanicals used as a food or beverage, such as chocolate, cocoa, tea, spinach, rhubarb, etc., contain an ingredient called *oxalic acid,* a substance which interferes with calcium utilization, while some contain caffeine or

other stimulants. Alfalfa herb tea is said to possess no un-
friendly components and may be given to children and
adults of all ages. It is considered particularly good for
nursing mothers who must abstain from beverages containing caffeine. It is often regarded as an ideal beverage for
the aged because of its excellent nutritive elements and
the fact that it is so easily assimilated. Many people employ alfalfa herb tea as an excellent substitute for coffee
or ordinary tea. Some prefer to sweeten it with honey.

AMARANTH
(Amaranthus hypochondriacus)

Synonyms: Prince's Feather, Pile Wort, Lady Bleeding,
Red Cock's Comb.

This is an annual herb with an upright stem from 3 to
4 feet high. It has bright reddish-purple, clustering
flowers of a plume-like form, and is grown as an orna-
mental plant in the gardens of the Middle States.

In folklore, this flower is regarded as the symbol of immortality. The name is taken from the Greek *amarantos*
meaning "incorruptible." It was the practice among the
Greeks to spread the flowers of amaranth over the graves
of the dead to demonstrate their belief in the immortality
of the soul.

Milton expresses his sentiments about the amaranth in
the following lines.

> Their crowns inwove with Amaranth and gold;
> Immortal Amaranth, a flower which once
> In Paradise, fast by the tree of life,
> Began to bloom.

Moore writes that amaranth was used in the East for
decorating the hair, and Homer mentions that the people

of Thessaly wore crowns of amaranth at the burial of Achilles.

Medicinal Use of Amaranth

The wild plant is believed to possess more medicinal properties than the cultivated. Amaranth contains a generous amount of vitamins and minerals, and was used in the place of spinach during the Middle Ages.

For centuries the plant was employed as a remedy for profuse menstruation. The early herbalists also employed it in the treatment of diarrhea and dysentery.

Dr. O. Phelps Brown wrote an account of the herb in *The Complete Herbalist* (1865) in which he stated that the plant was an astringent, and said: "The decoction drank freely is highly useful in severe menorrhagia (profuse menstruation), in diarrhea, dysentery, etc." He also mentioned that it was used externally as a wash for ulcerated conditions of the mouth.

A medical herbal of the 20th century[1] also classified the herb as an astringent: "This herb is most noted as an effectual cure for profuse menstruation for which purpose a tea is to be drunk freely, four or five times a day. It is an astringent, and as such, it is useful in bowel complaints."

Potter's New Cyclopaedia of Botanical Drugs and Preparations cites the value of amaranth both as an internal and external medicine. For internal use it is given as follows:

> Medicinal Use: Astringent. Highly recommended in menorrhagia, diarrhea, dysentery, . . . The decoction is taken in wine-glassful doses.

AVOCADO

Avocados are native to Mexico and Central America,

[1] *Encyclopedia of Health and Home.*

and were grown long before the discovery of the New World. The Spanish found them being extensively used by the Aztecs and other natives as an important article of the diet. It was not until the last century, however, that the trees were successfully established in the United States. They were brought from Mexico and planted in Florida in 1833 by Henry Perrine, a prominent horticulturist. Later, in 1871, they were introduced into California.

The Health Value of the Avocado

Avocados have a high content of protein and are often used in parts of Mexico and Central America as a substitute for meat. They are also very rich in unsaturated fatty acids and for this reason Dr. Wilson C. Grant, of the Veterans' Administration Hospital, Coral Gables, Florida, and the University of Miami School of Medicine decided to find out if they would reduce the cholesterol of the blood in selected patients.[2]

Ranging in age from 27 to 72, sixteen male patients were put on control diets to determine as closely as possible the normal cholesterol level of their blood. As a substitute for part of their dietary fat consumption they were given ½ to 1½ avocados each day. Twice a week measurements of their blood were taken. Eight of the sixteen patients showed marked decreases in total serum cholesterol from 8.7 to 42.8 percent. Eight experienced no change; however, one patient was very prone to high cholesterol content in the blood while three others were diabetics. In all who took part in the test, the cholesterol level either went down or stayed the same.

CALAMUS
(Acorus calamus)
Synonyms: Sweet Flag, Myrtle Flag, Sweet Cane, Sweet Root, Sweet Rush, Sweet Grass.

[2] *Prevention Magazine,* October 1960.

Calamus, or sweet flag in the domestic medication of India, is recorded from earliest times. Ainslie in his *Materia Medica of Hindoostan,* 1813, states that in consequence of its great value in the bowel complaints of children, a severe penalty was placed on the refusal of any druggist to open his door at night to sell sweet flag when demanded. The antiquity of its use is shown from the fact that it was one of the constituents of the ointment Moses was commanded to make for use in the Tabernacle (Ex. 30:23), while the prophet Ezekiel (27:19) says of the commerce of Tyre, ". . . . *bright iron, casia, and calamus, were in thy market.*" Theophrastus mentioned calamus, and Celsus, nearly two thousand years ago, referred to it as a drug from India. From its tropical home, calamus has spread until it is found now in all temperate climates suitable for its growth.

Medicinal Use of Calamus

Dr. Swinburne Clymer[3] gives the following account of the herb:

> When every known remedy has failed to stop the eruction of the awful burning water from the stomach into the throat, a small piece of calamus slowly chewed and the juice swallowed, nearly always will bring prompt relief. Those suffering from this irritating condition will do well to keep a piece of calamus root always at hand and to chew it regularly until the condition of the stomach which produces this is overcome . . .
>
> Children suffering continually from gas in the stomach should be given a weak tea of it at regular intervals.

[3] *Nature's Healing Agents.*

CANCERILLO[4]

Growing in the jungles of Costa Rica is a milkweed plant which bears multi-colored flowers. The plant is referred to as *cancerillo* by natives inhabiting the jungle villages of Central America who have used the plant for ages as a remedy for cancers, warts, and similar growths.

Samples of "cancerillo" were submitted to the University of Wisconsin by Professor J. A. Saenz Renauld, of the University of San Jose. At Wisconsin, a team of scientists headed by Professor S. Morris Kupchan which has already tested thousands of varieties of other plants, found an active ingredient in "cancerillo" that destroys human cancer cells in a test tube.

Whether or not the "cancerillo" extract will prove effective in curing cancers in living human beings is not yet known.

The New York *Herald Tribune* draws attention to the fact that "cancerillo's" active ingredient appears to be a chemical called *calotropin* which has been known to scientists for a long time. However they did not know that it could destroy cancer cells.

When they examined the molecule of *calotropin,* they found that it was similar to those of extracts from plants of the Dogbane[5] family, which are used as heart tonics. *Vinca rosea* (a species of Periwinkle) is also related to the Dogbane family and produces a drug which has been found effective in destroying cancers in humans and animals. Canadian Hemp is another plant related to the Dogbane family. It is regarded as a heart stimulant and also contains two active properties which destroy cultured cancer cells.

[4] *Fate Magazine,* June 1965 (Evanston, Ill.: Clark Publ. Co.).

[5] The common name for the family of shrubs, herbs and trees classified as *apocymacae.*

CHERRY TREE

The cherry tree is of Asiatic origin, and Pliny mentions that it was brought to Italy about 68 B.C. by Lucullus. It is cultivated extensively and thrives best in temperate climates. The wild species which is found in many countries produces excellent wood for cabinet work and furniture.

All parts of the cherry tree have been used as folk-medicine. In some countries a tea was made from the bark and employed as an astringent. The Indians prepared a decoction of the root which they used for various disorders. Cherry gum dissolved in wine is still a favorite in many lands for the relief of coughs.

Modern Research on the Cherry[6]

In the Texas Reports on Biology and Medicine, Vol. 8, Fall 1950, Ludwig Blau, M.D., writing on "Cherry Diet Control for Gout and Arthritis," proposed a large cherry intake as effective in the treatment of these diseases. We are told that the blood uric acid in 12 cases of gout dropped to its usual average and "no attacks of gouty arthritis have occurred on a non-restricted diet in all 12 cases, *as a result of eating about one half-pound of fresh or canned cherries per day.*" In giving the details concerning 3 of these cases, he shows that relief was brought about by the eating of either fresh Black Bing varieties, or canned cherries, sour, black, or Royal Anne. Only the juice was taken in one case and the effectiveness proved to be about equal.

An article appeared eight years later in the *Food Field Reporter* for November 10, 1958 on canned cherry juice relieving arthritis. The *Reporter* tells us that Reynolds Brothers, Incorporated, at Sturgeon Bay, Wisconsin, cited

[6] *The Complete Book of Food and Nutrition,* J. I. Rodale (Emmaus, Pa.: Rodale Books, Inc.).

new evidence that gouty arthritis, gout and similar ailments may be relieved by drinking canned cherry juice. It was reported that the cherry juice was tested daily by a number of Sturgeon Bay residents who gave their cooperation. The president of the firm that sold the cherry juice said that "Outstanding results were reported." He adds that the sale of his product has increased in Texas since the article appeared there, connecting cherry juice with arthritic relief.

The *Food Field Reporter* says:

> Today, there is no definite scientific data on just how the juice aids in relieving pain caused by diseases where improper balance of calcium is evident. However, it is believed that it may be the pigment in the cherries that brings relief.

CLOVES
(*Eugenia caryophyllata*)

Synonym: Clavos.

This small tree inhabits the Molucca Islands (once known as the Clove Islands), and the southern part of the Philippines. It is an evergreen with a pyramidal form and bears a succession of beautiful rose colored flowers throughout the year. The green leaves when bruised are highly fragrant and the flowers emit a strong penetrating odor.

Cloves Unknown to the Ancients

It appears that cloves were unknown to the ancients. They were introduced into Europe by the Arabians and distributed by the Venetians. After the southern passage to India was discovered, the spice trade of cloves passed into the hands of the Portuguese, and was subsequently wrested from them by the Dutch. The Dutch adopted a monopolizing policy of commerce and destroyed all of the clove trees throughout the Moluccas except on the islands of Ternate and Amboina which they kept under constant protection. However, in spite of their vigilance, a French governor named Poivre succeeded in the year 1770 in obtaining plants from the Moluccas and introduced them into colonies under his control. Fives years later the clove tree was introduced into the the West Indies and Cayenne; in Sumatra in 1803, and Zanzibar in 1818. In 1872 the clove orchards of Zanzibar were almost entirely destroyed by a hurricane, but were later replanted. Today, approximately three-fourths of the world's supply of clove is grown in Zanzibar and the neighboring island of Pemba. In 1952, 1,867,560 pounds of unground cloves were shipped into the United States from British East Africa, Madagascar and Ceylon. Clove oil, in the amount of 456,816 pounds, entered this country in the same year from British East Africa, Madagascar, Netherlands and France.

Part of the Plant Used as Cloves

The part of the plant employed under the name of cloves is the unexpanded flower buds. They are not gathered until the tree is about six years old. At first the buds are white, then become green, then bright red, at which point it becomes necessary to gather them immediately. They are either picked by hand or the trees are beaten with bamboos and the falling buds are caught. It is said that in the Moluccas the buds are immersed in boiling water, then exposed to smoke and artificial heat. In Zanzibar, Pemba, the West Indies and Cayenne they are dried by solar heat.

Cloves as Medicine

Cloves have been used as a tea, or in the form of a

powder, as a home remedy for the relief of gas, nausea or vomiting. The oil is well known as a domestic remedy for the relief of toothache. Herbalists as well as many of the old time family physicians regarded cloves particularly as astringent, stimulant and carminative. Dr. Fox, in his book *The Working Man's Model Family Botanic Guide*[7] describes their value in the following way:

Cloves are a stimulant and aromatic astringent, and useful to allay nausea and vomiting, to relieve flatulent colic, to improve digestion, as a healthy stomachic, and as an astringent, also valuable as an ingredient in compounds for the cure of diarrhea and dysentery. A little powdered cloves is often combined with other medicines to prevent them from griping or producing sickness at the stomach. Dose of the powder, from 10 to 20 grains.

The Dispensatory of the United States of America, 25th Edition, lists the use of clove *oil* as follows:

Uses. By virtue of its local irritant effect clove oil stimulates peristalsis and has frequently been employed in the treatment of flatulent colic. It also possesses some local anesthetic action, being a favorite remedy for toothache; for this purpose a small pledget of cotton is saturated with oil and inserted into the carious cavity. It is a powerful germicide, about eight times as strong as phenol, but is not frequently used, except by dentists, because of its irritant properties. Eugenol, the principal constituent of clove oil, has been used internally in daily doses of 3 ml. (approximately 45 minims) as an antiseptic antipyretic; it has also been used in treating patients with gastric or duodenal ulcers by instillation into the stomach . . . Little, however, is known of its physiological action. According to Leubuscher (Wien. med.

[7] Reprinted 1963 by Health Research, Mokelumne Hill, Calif.

Bl., 1889), it is a feeble local anesthetic. Landis (Therap. Gaz., 1909, 33, 386) used clove oil as a stimulant expectorant in tuberculosis and bronchiectasis with good results.

ECHINACEA

(*Echinacea angustifolia*)

Synonym: Coneflower.

There are four species of echinacea which inhabit the central and eastern parts of the United States. The flowers of the medicinal variety range in color from deep purple-red through rose-pink to white.

Echinacea, like cinchona, cocoa and other plants, was first used by the aborigines. The American Indians also employed it.

Conditions Affecting the Medicinal Properties in Herbs

It is well known that the medicinal properties of herbs are influenced in various degrees by conditions prevailing in different localities, i.e., soil, climate, etc., as well as the method of curing and drying. The quality of echinacea is strongly influenced by such conditions. In some localities it seems almost devoid of medicinal value. From favorable regions, the properties may be ruined by a careless process of curing. Examples of the importance of proper aging and curing may be realized in considering several common articles such as apple cider, grapes, tea, etc. Through carelessness, apple cider or wine may turn to vinegar. By special drying methods, grapes are made into raisins.

Medicinal Use of Echinacea

The first mention of echinacea in a medical journal appeared as a note by Dr. John King in 1887. Its use by other physicians quickly followed and the plant was lauded as an excellent blood purifier and alterative. In 1910, Dr. Neiderkorn wrote that: "Echinacea is a corrector of the depravations of the body fluids . . ."

Echinacea has not been without opposition, as the enthusiasm of a few physicians apparently led to exaggerated statements of its power in some directions. To give the conclusions of an observing physician whose knowledge of echinacea was gained in bedside practice, the following extracts are reprinted from the conservative writings of Dr. W. H. Felter, a former Therapeutic Editor of the *American Dispensatory:*

> *Internal.* Echinacea is stimulant, tonic and depurative; it is in a lesser degree anesthetic and antiputrefactive. The necessity for remedies that favor the elimination of caco-plastic material is most marked when one is treating diseases which show a depraved condition of the body and its fluids. Such, a remedy for "blood depravation" if we may use that term, is Echinacea. No satisfactory explanation for its action has ever been given, and that a simple drug should possess such varied and remarkable therapeutic forces and not be a poison itself is an enigma, still to be solved, and one that must come as a novelty to those whose therapy is that of heroic medicines only. If there is any meaning in the term alterative, it is expressed in the therapy of Echinacea. For this reason, a most excellent medicine has been lauded extravagantly and came near to damnation through the extravagant praises of its admirers.
>
> Echinacea is a remedy for autoinfection, and where the blood stream becomes slowly infected either from within or without the body. Elimination is imperfect, the body tissues become altered, and there is developed within the fluids and tissues septic action with adynamia, resulting in boils, carbuncles, cellular tissue inflammations, abcesses and other septicemic processes. It is therefore a drug indicated by the *changes manifested in a disturbed balance of the fluids of the body, resulting in tissue alteration—be the cause in-*

fectious by organisms, or devitalized morbid accumulations, or alterations in the blood itself.

It is not by any means a cure-all, but so important is its action that we are inclined to rely largely on it as an auxiliary remedy . . .

External Use. Echinacea is stimulant, deodorant, and anesthetic. Alcoholic preparations applied to denuded surfaces cause considerable burning discomfort, but as soon as the alcohol is evaporated a sense of comfort and lessening of previous pain is experienced. Its deodorant powers are remarkable, especially when applied to foul surfaces, carcinomatous ulcerations, fetid discharges from the ears, and in gangrene, much to the comfort of the sick and the attendants. Echinacea is useful as an application where decay is imminent or taking place, reparative power is poor, and the discharges sanious and unhealthy . . .

For ordinary stings and bites not venomous its internal as well as external use is advisable.

Used by spray it is effective to remove stench and to stimulate repair in tonsillitis . . .

Dr. Felter adds that echinacea is sometimes valuable in the treatment of eczema or chilblains. He mentions further that a special preparation composed of echinacea, asepsin, and tincture of myrrh was found effective as a mouth wash for bleeding gums, halitosis, etc.

Information on Echinacea from Other Sources

Eric Powell, N.D., Ph.D., M.N.I.M.H., of England, considers echinacea as one of the best herbal alteratives.[8] He states further that, "We have only recently discovered that it has a marked affinity for the prostrate gland, and may be used for enlargement and weakness of this organ."

Dr. Powell mentions the case of an elderly patient with

[8] *Health From Herbs Magazine*, October 1957.

enlarged prostate who had great difficulty in passing urine. He says, "Five drops of the combined tinctures of echinacea and sabal (saw palmetto) normalized the gland in three months. I was particularly pleased with the result in this case owing to his age, for he was over seventy!"

Dr. Swinburne Clymer regards echinacea as "the one true alterative."

Potter's New Cyclopaedia of Botanical Drugs and Preparations classifies the herbs as both alterative and antiseptic.

HAWTHORN
(Crataegus oxycantha)
Synonyms: English Hawthorn, May Bush, Haw.

This small thorny tree or shrub is found in Asia and Europe but is naturalized in many areas of North America. It bears crimson flowers and produces a red fruit (hawthorn berries) with yellow pulp which remains on the tree after the leaves drop off in autumn. The botanical name is taken from the word *kratos,* meaning strength, in reference to the hardness and strength of the wood, and *akantha,* meaning a thorn.

According to Christian legend, the Crown of Thorns was believed to be made of hawthorn; therefore, the herb was thought to possess miraculous healing properties. Other Christian legends state that the staff of Joseph of Arimathea which sprouted when thrown to the ground, was none other than hawthorn. In ancient Greece, the herb was used as a marriage torch, while in Rome it was considered a potent charm against sorcery and witchcraft. The leaves were placed in the cradles of new-born babies to invoke a special blessing and protection. The Greek bride was sometimes adorned with a sprig of hawthorn and the bridal altar decked with its blossoms. This practice was believed to secure a beautiful and blessed future for both bride and groom.

Hawthorn as a Medicine

According to old records, an Irish doctor in the last century had been obtaining good results when administering a "secret remedy" to heart patients. It was years before it was discovered that he had used a medicine made from hawthorn berries. Later, many herbalists and a few doctors began successfully treating certain types of heart disorders with this herbal medicine.

In 1899, an American physician, Dr. Lyle, mentioned the use of hawthorn in his *Physio-Medical Therapeutics, Materia Medica and Pharmacy*. He wrote: "The fruit of this shrub is highly commended as a heart tonic and by some is thought to be superior to Cactus in angina, oedema, regurgitation, enlargement, fatty degeneration. It influences the general system much as an alterant and is valuable in inflammatory rheumatism."

Modern Research on Hawthorn

In recent years, hawthorn has come under scientific investigation. Ullsperger (Pharmazie, 1951, 141) isolated a yellow substance from English hawthorn and found that it produced dilation of the coronary vessels. It was reported by Fasshauer (Deutsche med. Wchnschr., 1951, 76, 211) that one hundred heart patients requiring continuous therapy were given the liquid extract and the results were generally beneficial. Marked subjective improvement was noted in patients with mitral stenosis and patients with heart diseases of old age. In other patients, digitalis could be either temporarily discontinued or considerably reduced when hawthorn extract was administered.

PEPPERMINT
(*Mentha piperita*)

Synonyms: Brandy Mint, Lammint.

Mints, such as peppermint, spearmint, horse-mint, etc., are found throughout Europe, North Africa and Asia Minor. These have been popular herbs from earliest times and "tithes of mint" are mentioned in the New Testament. They have long been valued for their culinary and medicinal properties, and are used as an ingredient in mint sauces, mint jelly, sherbets, candies, etc., and are commonly prepared as teas for indigestion.

Peppermint is presently grown on a commercial basis in North America, eastern Asia, and Europe. Most of the peppermint produced in the United States comes from the Pacific Northwest, Michigan, and northern Indiana.

How to Distinguish Peppermint from Spearmint

Confusion often arises in distinguishing peppermint from spearmint; however, there are a few features of difference that can be easily noted. For example, the leaves of peppermint are broader, shorter, and a much darker shade of green than spearmint. In chewing the leaves of peppermint a pronounced cooling sensation is experienced when inhaling the breath while no such marked effect is noticed in chewing the leaves of spearmint.

Medicinal Use of Peppermint

Peppermint has been used for ages as a home remedy for indigestion, nausea, gas pains, or to modify the griping effects or bitter taste of other medicines. The Indians used peppermint tea as a vermifuge, while the early settlers employed it for dyspepsia. In Jamaica, peppermint tea is used for colic. In early times the mints were placed in the baths as it was believed they imparted a calming and strengthening effect to the nerves and muscles.

The Dispensatory of the United States of America,
25th Ed., lists the use of peppermint *oil* as follows:

> *Uses.* Peppermint oil possesses the physiological
> actions and therapeutic effects of menthol; it is, how-
> ever, more irritant locally. It has been preferred for
> internal use because of its more pleasant taste. It is
> generally regarded as an excellent carminative (Sa-
> poznik, J.A.M.A., 1935, 104, 1792) and gastric
> stimulant, and is still widely employed in flatulence,
> nausea, and gastralgia. In a study on human beings
> Van Liere and Northrup concluded it had no per-
> ceptible effect of the emptying time of the stomach
> (J. Pharmacol., 1942, 76, 38). Heinz (Therap. Halb-
> montash., April 1, 1920) claimed that it is an active
> cholagogue and recommended its use in gallstones.
> As a local application for coryza [9] it was used in
> strengths of from 0.5 to 1 per cent in liquid petro-
> latum or olive oil. Incorporated into a lozenge it has
> been used as a pleasant and efficient antiseptic and
> anesthetic in pharyngitis. For internal administration
> it may be dispersed in sugar and then given in aqueous
> solution, or more commonly in the form of the spirit.
> It is popular as a flavoring agent.

Peppermint Remedies

Drs. Wood and Ruddock wrote of the medicinal value
of the mints, and stated that relief follows almost immediately when oil of peppermint is applied to a burn. They
also considered peppermint effective in the following disorders:

> *Diarrhea. Essence* of peppermint properly admin-
> istered is one of the surest, as well as the simplest,
> remedies for this complaint. A bottle of peppermint

[9] Acute inflammation of the mucous membranes of the nasal
cavities.

should be kept in the medicine case of every family. As soon as an attack of diarrhea comes on, drop 15 drops of *essence* of peppermint in a teacupful of hot water, and sip with a spoon as hot as can be borne. Repeat the dose every three hours until cured.

Flatulent colic. Add one drop of the oil of peppermint to a half glass of hot water and drink as hot as possible. It is seldom necessary to repeat the dose as one will usually give almost immediate relief.

Nervous Sick Headache. To a teacupful of water add one teaspoonful of the *essence* of peppermint; saturate a cloth with it and apply to the head and temples. For many persons this will give very quick relief. As soon as the cloth becomes dry, wet the cloth again.

Seasickness. Give the *essence* of peppermint, particularly after free vomiting has occurred. To one teacupful of hot water add a teaspoonful of the *essence;* sweeten and take a swallow occasionally. If made warm each time, it will probably be more effective.

PERIWINKLE
(Vinca rosea)

Synonyms: Twinkles, Bright Eyes, Purity, Little Pinkie.

There are several varieties of periwinkle which are erect or trailing herbs. The one we are considering here is known botanically as *Vinca Rosea,* and is an erect, tender, tropical plant which is cultivated in green houses.

In floral language the periwinkle is regarded as representing sincere and unalterable friendship. In some countries the flowers are sent as presents between lovers and friends to acknowledge the pleasure of happy associations.

Periwinkle has been used by the natives in South Africa for many years as a remedy for diabetes. Considerable notice appeared in the London and South African press when a registration officer in Durban was reputedly cured after two months' treatment with the herb.

Scientific Research

A remarkable article written by Fred L. Shaw, Jr. appeared in *Drug Topics*, July 27, 1964. According to the article, it was reported to the American Society of Pharmacognosy at their fifth annual meeting that renewed emphasis in scientific plant research has resulted from the success doctors have had in prolonging the lives of cancer patients with two oncolytic agents derived from the periwinkle plant. Eli Lilly and Company markets the two drugs: vinblastine sulfate as *"Velban"* and vincristine sulfate as *"Oncovin."* We are further informed that, "Vinblastine is presently used in the treatment of generalized Hodgkin's disease and choriocarcinoma resistant to other therapy, and vincristine is indicated only in the treatment of acute leukemia in children. However, both drugs are under continual study for their efficacy in other types of cancer."

The article states that almost 200 researchers from our own country as well as abroad are meeting at the American Society of Pharmacognosy to discuss the periwinkle alkaloids and other potential derivatives of the plant and its botanical relatives. Dr. Emil Frei III of the National Cancer Institute said that the two drugs from the periwinkle plant represent an important advance in cancer therapy. He added that this discovery has created a strong impetus to search for oncolytic agents in the plant kingdom. Dr. Gordon H. Svoboda of Eli Lilly and Company, the 1963-1964 President of the American Society of Pharmacognosy, supports the views of Dr. Frei, and agrees that the anti-cancer alkaloids discovered in the periwinkle plant have greatly stimulated plant research. He has reported that some 50 alkaloids have been isolated from the periwinkle to date.

According to the article, "One fascinating report obliquely suggested that one could grow one's own Vinca rosea in one's own backyard." In growing some of these horticultural varients of the periwinkle for their pharmacognosal studies, Dr. Irene M. Hilinski, of the University of Pittsburgh, detailed some of the difficulties she and her fellow researchers overcame.

The white and "dwarf" varieties of the plant grown from seeds of Indian origin showed a "limited degree of activity" according to the researchers. Extracts from plants apparently devoid of any pharmacologic activity were those with pink and bluish-pink flowers and the white flowers with red "eyes." It appears that Dr. Hilinski's group of scientific gardeners did very well in spite of these frustrations. Enough usable material was harvested to enable them to prepare extracts which proved valuable against certain types of leukemia in mice.

RED RASPBERRY
(Rubus strigosus)

This is a shrubby plant native to America and the northern parts of Europe and Asia. It is extensively cultivated in many parts of the world as a garden fruit. The ripened fruit is used in making jellies, jams, desserts and liquors.

Medicinal Value

This plant has been considered valuable for many years, particularly as an agent in relieving the painful spasms of childbirth. Early in the century, Dr. Fox wrote the following account:

RED RASPBERRY LEAVES—(Rubus strigosus)
Astringent and Tonic

The leaves and the roots are the parts used. A strong infusion is useful in looseness of the bowels and summer complaint of children; it is an excellent remedy in painful and profuse menstruation, and to regulate the labour pains of women in childbirth. A teacupful of strong red raspberry leaf tea, in which the juice of an orange has been pressed, taken three times a day during the last month of pregnancy, will render labour easy when the hour of parturition has arrived.

Recently, other physicians have also called attention to the healing properties of red raspberry leaves. Dr. Kirschner states:[10]

Herbalists have long prescribed raspberry leaf tea during pregnancy. Medical men laughed at this "superstition." Then came the confession by a woman physician, Violet Russell, M.D., who wrote in the London medical journal *Lancet:* "Somewhat shamefacedly I have encouraged expectant mothers to drink this infusion . . . In a good many cases, labor has been easy and free from muscular spasm."

Dr. Kirschner explains that, "During confinement, a pint of raspberry leaf tea is taken daily. Ordinary dosage is 10 to 20 ounces of hot tea made from an ounce of dried leaves steeped in 20 ounces of boiling water." He adds, "Sweeten with honey."

In the book *Herbs and the Fountain of Youth* [11] we find the following information:

Red Raspberry Leaves. A good source of vitamins A, B_1, C, G and E. They are rich in calcium, phosphorus, iron and an unknown factor which prevents miscarriage. I know of several cases where this was proved beyond a doubt. A woman had four

[10] *Nature's Healing Grasses.*

[11] Claudia V. James (Edmonton, Alta., Canada: Amrita Books) 1965.

miscarriages and despaired of ever bearing a child. Several doctors told her that she could never become a mother. On advice given by close members of my family she took to drinking raspberry leaf tea every morning during pregnancy. She gave birth to a lovely girl, and in eighteen months she had another. The labor in both cases was practically painless. Canadian women would do well to make a special note of this as more Canadian women die in childbirth than any other civilized country.

Potter's New Cyclopaedia of Botanical Drugs and Preparations carries this notation:

> Dr. Thompson and Dr. Coffin recommended the drinking of the Raspberry Leaf tea by pregnant females for giving strength and rendering parturition easy and speedy. It should be taken freely before and during confinement . . .

ROSE HIPS AND ACEROLA BERRIES

Rose Hips

Rose hips are the fruit of the rose after the flower has bloomed and the petals have fallen, just as the cherry is the fruit of the cherry blossom. Rose hips are orange in color when not quite ripe; dark red when overripe; and bright red when fully ripe. The ancient Greeks in the time of Homer made a food of rose hips and a thousand years before Christ, the hips were referred to as the Food of the Gods. "Gods" were believed to be men who lived so close to nature that she whispered all her secrets to them.

The Nutritive Properties of Rose Hips

During World War II the governments of England, Sweden and Norway were faced with a serious shortage of vitamin C when they were unable to get fresh citrus imports. Knowing that they must protect the health of their people by supplying them with a source of vitamin C, they began a research of the properties of their local botanicals. After testing many wild fruits and plants, they discovered that rose hips contained an astonishing amount of vitamin C, ranging from 10 to 100 times greater than any other known food. The hips were used in the form of teas, soups. purées, etc.

Rose hips are still a favorite nutritious food in European countries today. In addition to their high content of vitamin C, they also contain vitamins A, E, B₁, B₂, niacin, K, P, and calcium, phosphorus and iron.

Species of Rose Hips

The hips from any healthy rose plant are used but garden varieties are said to be lower in vitamin C content than those of wild roses. Some species of wild roses have a higher content than other wild species. *Rosa laxa, Rosa rugosa, Rosa cinnamomea, Rosa acicularis* and *Rosa eddieii* are among the best in this regard.

Acerola Berries

In the tropics, the acerola is called the *Health Tree*. It is also known by a variety of other names such as Puerto Rican cherry, West Indian cherry, Barbados cherry, but more commonly as acerola berry. The fruit somewhat resembles the North American cherry but is actually a semi-tropical fruit known botanically as *Malpighia punicifolia.*

Scientific Investigation of the Acerola Berry

Scientific investigation has determined that acerola berries are the richest known source of vitamin C and also contain a good amount of other vitamins and nutritive elements. Scientists estimate that it would require about 50 pounds of fresh cabbage juice to yield as much vitamin C as found in only 6 ounces of acerola berries!

This semi-tropical fruit was discovered growing in Puerto Rico and plantations were cultivated to provide the people of that country with a natural food source of vitamin C. A new industry has consequently developed which not only furnishes the island with this nutritional food but also the world at large. The berries are supplied in the form of concentrated juices and as dehydrated juice in powdered form. The juice is blended with other fruit juices and is used with foods.

Recent Reports on Vitamin C

Although the value of vitamin C has already been mentioned elsewhere in this book, its importance to the health of the body is brought to the attention once again as research reports of over 100 medical teams have recently been cited in a publication entitled *The Key To Good Health—Vitamin C* by Fred Klenner, M.D., with Fred Bartz. A few excerpts from this report are given as follows:

Abstracts of published Medical Reports

There are probably 500 to 1,000 medical reports published on the use of vitamin C, in medicine. Observers the world over note its use as the basis of "tissue integrity." Again and again this is repeated. Some use the simile "it acts like mortar between bricks." Seldom is vitamin C used alone. Basic medicine is utilized first. As a supplement, C is only one of many important vitamins, minerals and enzymes, and other items that make up a complete, sound diet. The following summary of reports may be of interest to you. If you wish to read the original report, the file data is added for your information.

Abortions, habitual

Good results from the use of hesperidin and C.
Also used C, K and hesperidin.
S. Horoschak, Exper. Med. & Surg. 12:570-597, 1954.

Alcoholism

Intravenous administration of 1500 mg. of vitamin
C, 1000 mg. of vitamin B_1, doses of vitamin B_6 from
50 to 200 mgs. for delirium tremens or cases likely
to shortly become so. Repeated daily in smaller doses.
Sedation may be unnecessary. Rapid abatement of
symptoms.
J. S. Imrie, Brit. M. J. 2:428-30, Aug. 13, 1955.

Arteriosclerosis, ocular

Local arteriosclerosis and hemorrhages in the vitre-
ous are improved if 300 to 500 mgs. of vitamin C
and rutin are given daily. Chronic infection of the
cornea and ocular disturbances associated with vascular dysfunction are dealt with effectively with large
doses of vitamin C.
A. M. Yudkin.

Arthritis, rheumatic diseases and vitamin C

I have treated a number of rheumatic fever patients
with i.v. and oral doses of vitamin C from 1 to 10
grams daily. Recovery was routine in from three
to four weeks. No cardiac complications.

Those with incipient arthritis were given ascorbic
acid therapy and similar results achieved.

It seems to me that articular cartilaginous lesions
common to all rheumatic diseases are referable to
nutritional deficiency of vitamin C.

W. J. McCormick, M.D. Arch. Pediat. 70:107-112,
April 1955.

Cure for the common cold

For the common cold, usually three (3) 500 mg.

C tablets taken with fruit juice each hour for ten doses. Then four (4) C tablets every two hours around the clock will cure in 24 to 36 hours. If the cold is of the allergic rhinitis type, then one massive dose of C given intravenously (10 grams injected into the vein) followed with one of the antihistamines every 4 hours for six (6) times will do the job. Fred R. Klenner, M.D.

Edema, ocular

Edema of the macular region produced by vascular decompensation often responds more rapidly when 10 to 33 ounces of orange or grapefruit juice are given in addition to 500 mgs. of vitamin C daily for three or four days.
A. M. Yudkin, A. J. of Opth. 34:901-902, June 1951 (in Soc. Proc.).

Hypertension, cardiovascular and cerebrovascular diseases in the aged

Many illnesses in the aged may be prevented with an adequate vitamin C intake. Particularly cerebrovascular disease and heart disabilities incidence may be largely reduced. Supplements of rutin and vitamin C should be routine. Doses of 500 to 1000 mgs. daily may be given by mouth, but when speed of absorption is required due to some emergency, i.m. or i.v. administration recommended.
E. T. Gale, M. W. Thewlis, Geriatrics 8:80-87, Feb. 1953.

Fast relief from Prickly Heat

Relief from prickly heat within thirty minutes by administration of vitamin C in doses of 500 mgs. was reported by Dr. Robert L. Stern, Journ. A.M.A., 1/20/51 in the South Pacific Islands to troops stationed there during World War 2.

Stress and C, Preventing surgical shock

I found that surgeons employ ascorbic acid rou-

tinely before and after surgery . . . 500 mgs. by mouth
one hour before surgery to patients of average weight
reduced to a considerable extent traumatic shock . . .
500 mgs. orally is extremely useful in preventing
shock and postoperative weakness from tooth extraction . . . 500 mgs. or more to groups of coal miners
involved in a mining accident sustaining various
injuries increased shock resistance and measurably
improved their condition . . . intravenously administered doses of ascorbic acid 500 to 1,000 mgs. buf-
fered sterile solutions before and after in some 50
major operations "with excellent results."
H. N. Holmes, Ohio State M.J. 42:1261-1264, Dec.
1946 (abstr. J.A.M.A. 133:649, March 1, 1947).

Whooping cough

Ninety children with whooping cough were treated
with 500 mgs. of vitamin C, i.v. injection and orally,
daily, for one week. Every second day the dosage was
reduced by 100 mgs. The last dose was given continually until each child was completely recovered.
Children receiving C i.v. were well in 15 days, orally
in 20 days. The children treated with vaccine averaged
34 days duration. In three quarters of the cases when
vitamin C therapy was started in the catarrhal stage,
the spasmodic stage was wholly prevented.
J. C. de Wit, abstr. J.A.M.A. 144:879, Nov. 4, 1950.

Smoking reduces vitamin C in blood stream

A heavy smoker who inhales may show a decrease of
66% of vitamin C level in the blood stream. Addition
of nicotine to sample of whole human blood decreases
the vitamin C content by 24.4% to 31.6%.
A. Bourquin & E. Mussmano, Am. J. Digest. Dis.
20:75-77, March 1953.

Vitamin C Tablets Made from Rose Hips and Acerola Berries

During the process of making vitamin C tablets from

rose hips or acerola berries, the manufacturer generally allows some of the other natural substances from the original food to remain with the vitamin C. Depending on the preparations as stated on the labels, these may include the bioflavonoids and/or rutin, hesperidin, etc.

Vitamin C tablets made from rose hips or acerola berries are available from health food stores.

SLIPPERY ELM
(Ulmus fulva)
Synonyms: Rock Elm, Sweet Elm, Indian Elm, American Elm, Moose Elm, Red Elm.

The inner bark of slippery elm was an important medicine and food of the American Indians and pioneers. The Indians also used it to prevent fatty substances from becoming rancid. This was done by melting the fat of an animal with a piece of the bark and allowing the preparation to remain heated for a few minutes, then the fat was strained off. During the last century, Dr. C. W. Wright tested this Indian formula by following the same procedure with lard and butter, and found that rancidity was prevented for a long time.

As a healing agent, the Indians applied slippery elm bark in the form of a poultice for wounds, burns, etc. Internally, it was used as a tea, so that its soothing properties could reach the deep-seated delicate membranes of the throat as well as irritations of the stomach and intestines. The pioneers used it in the same way as the Indians and also employed the tea as a wash for chapped hands and face. As a food, the bark was powdered, mixed as a beverage and given to babies, the elderly, and those recuperating from illnesses.

The Gentle Action of Slippery Elm

Slippery elm is considered one of nature's finest demulcents, and is used for its ability to absorb noxious gases and neutralize stomach acidity. The powdered bark mixed with milk is said to be wholesome and nutritious. Because of its mucilaginous nature, its use insures an easy passage during the process of assimilation and elimination. Its action is so gentle that it can be retained by delicate stomachs when other foods are rejected. Many preparations of the powdered bark are manufactured and sold on the market as bland and nutritious foods.

Medical herbals invariably included information on the value and use of slippery elm. For example, Dr. Fox wrote:

> *Slippery elm bark.* It is a very valuable remedy employed chiefly in mucous inflammation of the lungs, bowels, stomach, kidneys and bladder, taken freely in the form of a mucilaginous drink. One ounce of the bark is simmered slowly in two pints of water down to one pint. It is very beneficial in diarrhea, . . . pleurisy, dysentery, coughs, . . . and sore throat. A tablespoonful of this powder boiled in milk, affords a nourishing diet for infants, preventing the bowel complaints to which they are subject. As a poultice, it is far superior to linseed meal, applied to ulcers, boils, and carbuncles.

The following information on slippery elm is taken from the *Dispensatory of the United States,* 25th Edition:

> Elm bark is an excellent demulcent, formerly extensively employed especially in the form of lozenges, to relieve irritation of the pharynx. A warm infusion was a popular folk remedy in the treatment of diarrheas, coughs, etc. This was prepared by stirring an ounce of the powdered bark in a pint of hot water, with which it forms a mucilage which was taken *ad libitum.*
>
> The bark was used also as an emollient application in cases of external inflammation. For this purpose the powder was made into a poultice with hot

water, or the bark itself applied, previously softened by boiling.

Note: The best quality of slippery elm bark can be folded lengthwise without breaking while inferior grades are brittle.

VEGETABLE OILS [12]

Heart disease is mankind's No. 1 killer. Recently, in one year alone, deaths from heart ailments rose to 916,000 in the United States, and over one million in Russia. In Britain, the death rate from this disease in ratio to the population is the highest in the world.

Through extensive research, American, British and Russian medical scientists have all agreed that the prime factor in preventing atherosclerosis (a type of arteriosclerosis or hardening of the arteries) is a cholesterol-lowering diet. They also believe that atherosclerosis is chiefly responsible for the steadily growing menace of coronary thrombosis. The findings of the three countries show that increased substitution of vegetable oils for animal fats in the diet is the best method of reducing the cholesterol level in the blood.

America

Mrs. Dorothy Revell, chief dietician of the Dakota Clinic says:

> An important principle involved in a cholesterol-lowering diet is the ratio between unsaturated and saturated fats in the daily intake. For every gram of saturated fat there should be two to three grams of unsaturated fat.
>
> Frequently where there is a high level of choleste-

[12] *Here's Health,* October 1961.

rol in the blood there is a deficiency of a fatty acid called linoleic acid, which must be supplied to the body from the outside to act as a transportation agent in carrying the cholesterol along the bloodstream.

Because of its high linoleic acid content and the fact that it is easily obtainable, corn oil is the preferred unsaturated fat. In my area, Mazola corn oil is readily available and economic to use for all forms of cooking—browning meat, grilling fish, baking cakes and cookies. For some of my patients, I recommend an ounce of corn oil to be taken first thing each morning as a good start to the day.

Britain

Dr. Hugh M. Sinclair, Fellow of the Magdalen College, and for many years Reader in Human Nutrition at the University of Oxford, was chairman at an important discussion on atherosclerosis. Dr. Sinclair has contributed an important part in the recent conclusions of modern heart specialists. In his own research he has repeatedly found that the substitution in the diet of corn and other vegetable oils for animal fats has a pronounced and undeniable cholesterol-lowering effect:

Dr. Sinclair says:

Processing and sophistication of foods have destroyed the unstable helpful fats we need which are present in such natural oils as unhydrogenated corn oil, and have created stable harmful fats. The harmful saturated fats are, the American Heart Association reported recently, present in considerable amounts in most cooking fats and margarines. The helpful highly unsaturated fats occur in vegetable seed oils such as corn oil, cotton seed and soybean oil.

Russia

Dr. V. Socolovsky gave a report at the Third Annual

Congress of Dietetics, held at Church House, Westminster. He revealed that over 500 Russians with coronary atherosclerosis had been subject to laboratory tests. The results enabled Dr. Socolovsky and his colleagues at the Academy of Medical Sciences for the U.S.S.R., Moscow, to recommend a diet in which one-third of the fats are oils having a high unsaturated fatty acid content for the treatment and prevention of coronary atherosclerosis. Dr. Socolovsky reports that: "Of the tested oils, corn and sunflower oils have the best cholesterol-lowering activity."

VIOLET
(Viola odorata)
Synonyms: Sweet Violet, Blue Violet.

There are many species of violet ranging in shades from deep blue through yellow to white. Some emit a strong and pleasant fragrance while others are odorless.

The common sweet violet is very popular, and is grown extensively in gardens. This flower figures prominently in European literature and even entered the political field of Napoleon's time. It was said to be the secret badge of his adherents during his absence.

The violet was a favorite of both the Romans and Greeks, and was the national flower of Athens. Orators endeavoring to win the favorable attention of the people addressed them as "Athenians crowned with violets." In Persia, the Mohammedans flavored their sherbets with violets, while Romans drank a perfumed wine made from the blossoms. It was also considered a love potion.

In the symbolic language of flowers, faithfulness is appropriated to the blue variety of violets, innocence or modesty to the white, and happiness to the yellow.

Research on the Violet [13]

[13] *Science Digest,* February, 1960.

Dr. Jonathan Hartwell, a chemist of the Cancer Institute of the National Institutes of Health, has spent many years gathering material on folk medicine as it pertains to cancer. He estimates that he has collected over 3000 pamphlets and books on the subject for handy reference when the merits of folk medicine are tested by scientists.

Dr. Hartwell says:

In the early Creole days in Louisiana, the juice of the May apple root was used to treat warts. Other records show that the Penobscot Indians used the same remedy for the same purpose. This is interesting because the Penobscots and the Creoles were widely separated.

And we have found that ancient Chinese treated tumors with herbs that were used also in Africa.

The violet plant, as far back as 500 B.C., was used in poultice form as a cure for surface cancer. It was used in 18th century England for the same purpose. And now only months ago—a letter from a farmer in Michigan tells me how he used the violet plant as a skin cancer remedy. When the remedy was tried on a cancerous mouse here at the Institute, we found that it did damage the cancer.

Now all these things present complex questions. We can't be sure the disease treated was really cancer. Scientific investigation should shed some light on this. Meanwhile, I am hoping that those who still have in their families, old records of folk remedies will send them in to us. In time we will try to check their efficacy.

conclusion

BIOCHEMIC RESEARCH HELPS us to appreciate the high value placed on plant medicine from the earliest periods of time. Nature has not lost her friendly touch and is demonstrating to us, just as she has demonstrated to former generations, the medicinal power of natural or herbal drugs. In fact, due to the combined efforts of our medical teams and their laboratory methods of plant analysis and experimentation, we of the present age may expect the botanicals to do much more for us than they did for our forefathers.

Botanical Renaissance?

In the book, *Nature's Remedies* [1] published in 1934, this timely bit of information was cited:

> Back to Grandma's medicine chest. This was the keynote of an address by Dr. Ivor Griffith, of the faculty of the Philadelphia College of Pharmacy and Science recently delivered before the New Jersey State Pharmaceutical Association. He says:
> "No one can convince me that grandmother's fresh drug infusions or old-fashioned teas of garden herbs

[1] Joseph E. Meyer, Indiana Botanic Gardens, Hammond, Ind., 1934.

had no special value. Too much neglected have been sage and chamomile, boneset and mullein, bitter apple and horse nettles, plantain and heal-all, liverwort and tansy, pumpkin seeds and mallow and a host of other herbs that have served the country for centuries with their ministrations.

"A host of drugs deserving a better destiny lie prematurely buried. In a mad scramble to squeeze out of the coal-tar barrel every available virtue, research has neglected the botanicals. There is a myriad of plant antidotes to pain waiting for proper appraisal. It is high time for a botanical renaissance."

Are we now entering that botanical renaissance called for by Dr. Griffith over 30 years ago? Every indication points to the fact that we are, as numerous medicines derived from plants are gradually achieving an honored place among the materia medica of modern man. As time goes by their number will undoubtedly increase, and from the many facts existing it does not seem unreasonable to speculate that in the future, freedom from every disease may possibly be found in the healing agents of the plant kingdom.

glossary

Alterative: A vague term to indicate a substance which alters a condition by producing a gradual change toward the restoration to health.

Anodyne: Eases pain.

Anthelmintic: Expels or destroys intestinal worms.

Antidote: Agents which counteract or destroy the effects of poison or other medicines.

Antiscorbutic: Counteracts scurvy.

Antiseptic: Destroys or inhibits bacteria.

Antispasmodic: Prevents or allays spasms or cramps.

Aphrodisiac: Stimulates the sex organs.

Appetizer: Stimulates the appetite.

Aromatic: Agents which emit a fragrant smell and produce a pungent taste. Used chiefly to make other medicines more palatable.

Astringent: Causes contraction of tissues.

Balsamic: A healing or soothing agent.

Bitter Tonic: Bitter tasting properties which stimulate the flow of saliva and gastric juice. Used to increase the appetite and aid the process of digestion.

Cardiac: Agents which have an effect on the heart.

Carminative: Expels gas from the stomach, intestines or bowels.

233

Cathartic: Causes evacuation from the bowels. There are different types of cathartics. Aperients or laxatives are mild and gentle in their actions. Purgatives are powerful and produce copious evacuations and are used only by adults afflicted with stubborn conditions.

Cholagogue: Increases the flow of bile and promotes its ejection.

Cordial: Invigorating and stimulating.

Counterirritant: Agents applied to the skin to produce an irritation for the purpose of counteracting a deep inflammation.

Demulcent: Soothing, bland. Used to relieve internal inflammations. Provides a protective coating and allays irritation of the membranes.

Depurative: A purifying agent.

Detergent: Cleansing.

Digestive: Aids digestion.

Diuretic: Increases the flow of urine. (Because of their soothing qualities, demulcents are frequently combined with diuretics when irritation is present.)

Emmenagogue: Encourages the menstrual flow.

Emollient: Emollients are used externally only. They are employed for their softening and soothing effect.

Expectorant: Induces expulsion or loosens phlegm of the mucous membranes of the nasal and bronchial passages.

Febrifuge: Reduces fever.

Galactagogue: Promotes the secretion of milk from the nursing breast.

Germicide: Destructive to germs.

Hypnotic: Induces sleep.

Invigorant: A strengthening agent.

Laxative: Causes the bowels to act.

Mucilaginous: Emits a soothing quality to inflamed parts.

Nervine: An agent which acts on the nervous system to temporarily relax nervous tension or excitement.

Nutrient or Nutritive: Nourishing.

Pectoral: Relieves affections of the chest and lungs.

Purgative: Causes copious evacuations from the bowels. Purgatives are more drastic than laxatives or aperients, and are generally combined with other agents to control or modify their actions. Used only by adults.

Reactivator: Restores to a state of activity.

Rejuvenator: An agent which imparts renewed vitality.

Restorative: Aids in the regaining of normal vigor.

Rubefacient: A substance used externally which causes redness and increased blood supply when rubbed into the skin.

Sedative: Calms the nerves.

Soporific: Induces sleep.

Specific: An agent or remedy that has a special effect on a particular disease.

Stimulant: Increases or quickens various functional actions of the system.

Stomachic: Substances which give strength and tone to the stomach. Also used to stimulate the appetite.

Sudorific: Produces copious perspiration.

Taeniafuge: Expels tapeworm.

Tonic: Invigorating and strengthening to the system.

Vermifuge: Expels or destroys worms.

Vesicant: Raises blisters.

EXPLANATION OF TERMS RELATING TO VARIOUS METHODS OF HERBAL PREPARATIONS

Decoctions: Decoctions are certain preparations made by boiling herbal substances in water for a considerable period of time. Hard materials such as roots, bark, seeds, etc., are usually prepared in this way as they require longer subjection to heat in order to extract their active principles. Generally 1 ounce of the botanical substance is placed in 1 pint of cold water. The container is then covered and the solution allowed to boil for one-half hour, after which it is then strained, cooled and ready for use. However, since some of the water boils away, many herbalists prefer to use 1½ pints of water so that when the boiling period has ended the decoction measures approximately 1 pint.

Extracts: Extracts are made in a variety of ways, depending on the best method by which the plant's properties may be obtained, such as high pressure, evaporation by heat, etc. Extracts are generally supplied by the various herb companies.

Infusions: Infusions are frequently called teas, and are generally prepared in the amount of 1 ounce of the plant substance to 1 pint of water. However, in some instances where the plant contains very active principles, less is sufficient. Usually the softer substances of the herb such as the blossoms, leaves, etc., are prepared as infusions. A pint of boiling water is poured over the herb, the container covered, and the solution allowed to steep (stand) for 15 minutes (stirring occasionally). When the steeping period has ended, the infusion is strained and used. Infusions are also frequently prepared by placing a teaspoonful of the plant substance in a cup and pouring boiling water over it. It is then covered with a saucer and allowed to steep for 15 minutes, after which it is strained and used. Sometimes a little honey is added to make the infusion more palatable. Infusions are never allowed to boil.

Poultices: Poultices are used to apply moist heat to draw or soothe. The fresh leaves are generally used, if available, and are crushed and steeped in boiling water for a short period of time. The leaves are then spread between two pieces of cloth and applied as hot as can be comfortably borne to the affected part, then covered with a dry cloth to retain the heat. A second poultice is prepared and used the moment the first one begins to noticeably lose the heat. The powdered herb is often used as a substitute for the fresh leaves. Enough of the powdered herb for several poultices is placed in a double boiler. Hot water is stirred into the powder until it attains the consistency of a paste. The paste is then spread between two pieces of cloth, applied and renewed several times.

Tinctures: Tinctures are spiritus preparations made with pure or diluted alcohol (not rubbing alcohol) or brandy, vodka, gin, etc. Tinctures are employed because some herbs will not yield their properties to water alone, or may be rendered useless by application of heat. In other instances, an herb will more readily impart its active principles when prepared as a tincture. Generally, 4 ounces of water and 12 ounces of spirits is mixed with 1 ounce of the powdered herb. The mixture is allowed to steep (stand) for 2 weeks, the bottle shaken thoroughly every night. After the steeping period has elapsed the clear liquid is strained off and the sediment discarded. The tincture is then bottled for use.

INDEX

238

Be healthy with Tandem

Hunza Health Secrets   **30p**
Renee Taylor

After two thousand years of almost complete isolation, the people of Hunza have revealed the way of eating, living and thinking that has substantially lengthened their lifespan and dramatically reduced susceptibility to most illnesses. You too can enjoy the benefits of the Hunza Health Diet, learn the basic disciplines of Hunza Yoga, and discover the life-enhancing power of increased mental and physical energy.

Instant Health the Nature Way   **30p**
Carlson Wade

How to put natural foods to work for you to fortify you against disease. A guide to the abundant variety of inexpensive everyday natural foods, with recipes and instructions for using them as your keys to good nutrition.

Macrobiotics   **25p**
Sakurazawa Nyoiti and William Dufty

More than a diet, Macrobiotics is a way of life which has been practised in the East for centuries. Based on the eating of whole grains, cereals, fish and selected vegetables, it has proved startlingly effective in treating a wide range of physical disorders as well as providing health and vitality.

The Rejuvenation Vitamin   **25p**
Carlson Wade

Vitamin E – the vitamin that can make you feel, look and think young for the rest of your life. Results indicate that Vitamin E may possess miracle restorative properties – and it is often lacking in the average diet. This book is devoted exclusively to this important vitamin, tells you from which foods you can find it, and helps you benefit from its remarkable qualities.

The Way of an Eagle

Dan Potter 30p

He came on a gleaming white motorcycle and some people
said that he looked like an eagle descending from the sky.
Was he a turned-on no-good looking for trouble, a rein-
carnated James Dean, or was he a messenger of peace and
goodwill? To some he was beauty and kindness, but to the
town hoodlums he was something they didn't understand,
instinctively feared, and had to destroy.

The Plasticine Man

Erika Maharg 25p

Bull Harrigan was many things to many people. A man for
all seasons, all reasons, every-woman's personal lover. He
had come to Spain to enjoy himself and he had neither the
will-power nor the inclination to refuse the women who
needed and wanted him. But they always demanded more
than he was prepared to give, sometimes more than he felt
he had. He wished they would stop trying to mould him into
what they wanted him to be.

Where's Poppa?

Robert Klane 25p

Some people have all the luck. Money and jobs and girls.
Especially girls. Gordon Hocheiser had the job, and the
money, but whenever he thought he was getting anywhere
near a girl, there was Momma. Momma - sitting in the
apartment, waiting for Poppa to come home, and seeing to
it that no one but herself laid hands on her son. Momma was
quite a woman!

Non-fiction in Tandem editions

Occult and the Supernatural in Tandem editions

Horror in Tandem editions

A Tree Grows in Brooklyn

Betty Smith

A novel which was hailed as a potential classic on its first appearance in America – "the best first novel I have seen ..." "a book worth getting excited about ..." "a superb feat of characterisation ..." "a profoundly moving novel ..." – this is the story of the Nolans, a devoted family, and their struggle to survive and rise above the squalor, poverty, and violence that surround their Brooklyn tenement home.

"A profoundly moving novel, and an honest and true one ... If you miss *A Tree Grows in Brooklyn* you will deny yourself a rich experience, many hours of delightful entertainment, and the pleasant tingle that comes from the discovery of a fresh, original and finished talent." *New York Times*

50p

The Raging Moon

Peter Marshall

The movingly tender love story of Bruce Pritchard, tough young Yorkshireman, and Annette Perel, a girl from a sheltered middle-class home. Thrown together from their widely differing backgrounds by misfortune, they fall in love. Despite the disapproval and lack of understanding of practically everyone around them, they retain their faith in themselves and their dreams for the future.

"His hero is malicious as well as brave, cocky as well as tender, but he has a passionate belief in life and love that gives the book a fiery urgency." *Times Literary Supplement*

25p

Name...

Address ....

Titles required ....

....

....

....

....

....

....

....

- -

The publishers hope that you enjoyed this book and invite you to write for the full list of Tandem titles which is available free of charge.

If you find any difficulty in obtaining these books from your usual retailer we shall be pleased to supply the titles of your choice — packing and postage 5p—upon receipt of your remittance.

WRITE NOW TO:
Universal-Tandem Publishing Co. Ltd.,
14 Gloucester Road,
London SW7 4RD